BEING FOUND

Healing the Very Young Through Relationship and Play Therapy

Dott Kelly

CHIRON PUBLICATIONS • ASHEVILLE, NORTH CAROLINA

© 2023 by Chiron Publications. All rights reserved. No part of this publication may be reproduced, stored in a retrieval system, or transmitted, in any form by any means, electronic, mechanical, photocopying, recording, or otherwise, without the prior written permission of the publisher, Chiron Publications, P.O. Box 19690, Asheville, N.C. 28815-1690.

www.ChironPublications.com

Interior and cover design by Danijela Mijailovic
Printed primarily in the United States of America.

ISBN 978-1-68503-107-7 paperback
ISBN 978-1-68503-109-1 hardcover
ISBN 978-1-68503-115-2 electronic
ISBN 978-1-68503-116-9 limited edition paperback

Library of Congress Cataloging-in-Publication Data

Names: Kelly, Dott, author.
Title: Being found : healing in the very young / Dott Kelly.
Description: Asheville, North Carolina : Chiron Publications, [2022] | Includes bibliographical references and index. | Summary: "The goal of the therapist is to find the child. When we have found the child, the child has also made an attempt at being seen. So there we are, face to face with the obstacles and disturbances between us. The child has made some kind of meaning-filled decision to come out and find us. In this space between, this joint, we are charged with holding still and listening for the many forms of nonverbal language the child may use to speak about their hurt. Premature efforts on our part may add static that pushes the child back, away from us. We will be tested in similar ways that the infant needed to test the integrity of an adult, when they cried out with their sharp and sudden needs. This book explores when something has gone wrong. But more so, ultimately it is about righting the relationship through the same trust the child requires at birth. When harm has occurred, the psyche endeavors to defend the self from annihilation by concealing it for the sake of protection within deep unconscious regions of the psyche. In this hidden place, the child suffers somatically and emotionally until the lost aspects can be safely found and re-embodied. In this, the child and the therapist enlist a third entity, the Us in the relationship, to reclaim lost aspects of psyche, or Self. Several chapters explore what us means to the child, with the child's expressions revealing this need for mutuality"-- Provided by publisher.
Identifiers: LCCN 2023003191 (print) | LCCN 2023003192 (ebook) | ISBN 9781685031077 (paperback) | ISBN 9781685031091 (hardcover) | ISBN 9781685031152 (ebook)
Subjects: LCSH: Play therapy. | Sandplay--Therapeutic use. | Psychic trauma in children--Treatment. | Child psychotherapy. | Therapist and patient.
Classification: LCC RJ505.P6 K37 2022 (print) | LCC RJ505.P6 (ebook) | DDC 618.92/891653--dc23/eng/20230417
LC record available at https://lccn.loc.gov/2023003191
LC ebook record available at https://lccn.loc.gov/2023003192

Contents

Introduction: Being Seen	1
Process and Content	3
Trauma in Early Development	3
Trauma's Limbic Overdrive	4
Co-transference in Attunement	6
Doing the Work	9
Technique and Process	10

Part I: Between Child and Therapist

Chapter 1 Delilah: Not Remembering	15
The Brain	17
The Between Location	22
Mapping Relationship in the Brain	25
Vigilance	28
Left Brain Development	33
Limbic System as the Third Brain	35
Dependency	37
Chapter 2 Annie and the Wolf: Remembering and Memory	43
Implicit and Explicit Memory	44
Therapeutic Helplessness	46
Fantasy as a Defense	49
Therapeutic Meaning Making	53
Memory Fragments	55
Remembering	56

Chapter 3 Jamal: Development and Trust	61
Creation of the Child	62
Trust as a Developmental Task	65
Gifts of the Limbic System	67
Trust Reprised	71
The Role of Language	73
The Child's Form of Knowing	77
Aggression	80
Chapter 4 Zack and "The Usman" - Back to the Beginnings	87
The Development in the Safety of Self	89
"Usman" Carrying the Relationship in Image	91
Batman and the Use of the Hero	93
Story in Image Form	96
Chapter 5 Orion: Implicit Memory	103
Parent as Regulator	104
Memory as Stored Up Feeling States	106
Relationship and Memory	109
The Child's Ways of Knowing	112

Part II: Stages of Treatment in Play Therapy

Chapter 6 Eric and the Cat	117
The Impact of Our Stories	118
The Therapist as the Tool	118
Therapeutic Road Signs	120
Decoding the Communications of Memory	124
Behind the Power Struggle	127
Chapter 7 Andy: Being Found	129
Compromised Trust	129
Instinctual Interactions between Mother and Baby	132
Healing From the Interior	133
Trauma From the Lack of Mirroring	135
Neglect in Me/Not-Me and Failure to Thrive	137
The Sameness of "Us"	143

Contents

Chapter 8 Andrea: Development Within the Therapy Setting — 147
   Early-Stage Treatment and Building Rapport — 148
   Second Phase of Treatment — 150
   Containment of the Unconscious in Play — 152
   Impairments From Trauma — 156
   Repair and Attunement — 159

Chapter 9 Mona: The Wounds of Abandonment — 163
   Aggression and Attachment — 163
   Silence and Neglect: Selective Mutism — 164
   "Don't Look at Me" and Neglect — 167
   Overwhelming Monsters: Implicit Memory — 168
   Metaphoric Expressions of Neglect — 172
   The Child's Interior Map — 177
   Therapeutic Tension — 178

Part III: Working in Transference: The Use of the Therapist

Chapter 10 Marnie: Co-transference — 183
   The Back and Forth of Co-transference — 184
   Feeling the Mutual "Us" Space — 187
   The Dangers of Transference Work — 188
   The "Remote Control" Metaphor — 189
   Therapeutic "Failure" — 191
   Reliance on the Child's Pace — 195

Chapter 11 Jake: Building the Self — 199
   Finding the Primitive Self through Image — 200
   The Willingness of the Therapist — 201
   Imagination — 203
   Jake's Internal War — 205
   The Toys as Alive Feeling States — 207
   Containing the Transference — 209
   Alchemical Images — 214
   Parent Consultations — 218
   The Fisher King Legend — 222
   Learning From the Child's Self — 226

Chapter 12 Ruthie: Challenges Between Us in Co-transference	229
Dynamics in the Co-transference	231
The Therapist's Self-Work	234
Requirement of Faith in the Child's Self	236
Implicit Memories Alive in the Present	237
Voices From the Unconscious	238
Limitations of Play Therapy	240
Working with Children Born Addicted	242
Working with Parent-Child Fused States	245
The Therapist's Wounds That Engage	249
Chapter 13 Clare: Transference and Imagination	251
Not Knowing How to Play	252
Being Found: The Work of Imagination	253
Access to the Unconscious Through Imagination	256
Imagination and Maria	257
Relational Space as Imaginal Space	261
The Therapist's Assignments	263
Imagination, Remembering and Being Remembered	264
Part IV: Supervision	
Chapter 14 Supervision: Faith and Doubt	269
Being Found as the Therapist Self	271
The Rawness of Hope	272
The Supervisor as Co-regulator	275
Faith and Doubt	277
False Knowing	279
The Strength of the Unconscious	282
Epilogue Rose: Remembering One's Self	287
The Child's Claimed Self	288
References	291
Index	295

I am grateful for my two children,
Jake and Delia, with their open-hearted faith
in living fully; and for the many children
whose lives have overlapped my own.

Disclaimer

All the children whose works are included in this book have been arduously veiled through the use of names, family environments, and situations. The dialogues of the children themselves have primarily remained intact, as these exchanges are at the heart of understanding how children make use of relationship, language, and symbols. Wherever possible, the chapters are amalgamates of children.

Use of the word "mother" is really about mothering, a dynamic that is not isolated to women. Mothering is about nurture. To mix and match "mothering" and "fathering" would have been distracting.

To maintain as much clarity as possible, I have interchanged masculine and feminine pronouns when the writing is apart from case studies.

Acknowledgements

This book's intent has grown throughout the years in the playrooms which were filled, hour after hour, with the work of children. I have relied on the stories from the children themselves in writing *Being Found*. I carried their question of "Will you remember me?" with me as I sat with these children and with many other therapists whose work with children sat between us. The children discovered their own ways to reach out and to try again to be understood. My deepest gratitude and respect to these young people and their families who put their trust in me.

Many adults have massaged this book into its physicality. Heather Macdonald was always available for wordsmithing, walking, and believing in this book. Mary Stowell checked my "temperature readings" for courage regularly, and brought me fine sweets for maintenance. Other friends who tirelessly encouraged each chapter into view include Janel Carlson, Virginia McIntyre, Gretchen Gubelman, Marian Birch, Mary Ann Smith, Barbara Putnam, and so many others who shared ideas and critical creativity. The play therapy work crew at Jumping Mouse Children's Center have been both inspirational and clarifying.

My editors, Anna Quinn and Elizabeth Baer, were crucial in setting the first drafts on their feet. And for years, Quen Zorrah and I travelled twice a month to our consultation group, creating new thoughts and linkages in our mutual work with children and families. Many of my ideas made first appearances in our shared vehicle. Thank you, Quen.

My appreciation to D.W. Winnicott, Ann Belford Ulanov, and Jessica Benjamin, whose efforts to articulate this mutual field within which we all exchange our truths worked inside me for the past 30 years, convincing me that I too could put words to the spaces between us all.

I come from a large family of a dozen, an intimate tribe who have challenged me from the get-go. Family members have read various chapters and drafts, and have been generous in their collected belief in me. We have always consciously held one another in the light. I love each of you.

I particularly owe gratitude to my long-time life partner, John, who believed in my dream of a book, and built me a shelter in which to set my experiences with children in therapy onto paper. And to my son and daughter Jake and Delia and my step-daughter Ellen, who are always present in me, and who offered jokes on the hard days, applause during the completed phases, and invaluable tech support, thank you.

Introduction: Being Seen

The goal of the therapist is to find the child. When we have found the child, the child has also made an attempt at being seen. So there we are, face to face with the obstacles and disturbances between us. The child has made some kind of meaning-filled decision to come out and find *us*. In this space between, this joint, we are charged with holding still and listening for the many forms of nonverbal language the child may use to speak about their hurt. Premature efforts on our part may add static that pushes the child back, away from us. And often the child must weave back and forth, taking a risk in being seen and then backing away again into the defenses that have served a purpose. We will be tested in similar ways that the infant needed to test the integrity of an adult, when they cried out with their sharp and sudden needs.

Trust is perhaps the lantern we carry as we move along, toward increasing tension and need from the child, toward what hurts. It is so difficult to witness pain in a child. The therapist's beliefs and fantasies might want to focus instead on the innocence, the beauty and the wonderment of children. These idealistic notions are brought down hard when we face a young child's pain.

Our own struggle with children's pain and what they may have suffered will push us, if we are not alert, to the fixing space. To crack open what this need may be, the word "fix" itself points to our struggle. To fix is "to put into a stable or unalterable form": "to preserve a specimen intact for microscopic study," "to correct or set right" (*Random House College Dictionary*). If we knew the danger in our attitudes, most of us would not go there. We are not about preserving anything for further research. If we move to a fix position, we tell the child that we are going into their perceptions and experiences to correct something that is not right. Children sense this intrusion before we quite know we have communicated it. When danger sends out alarms, the child tucks his head down in anxiety and even shame, and interrupts any wiring up, or longing to be found, by disappearing into the shadows once more. We have added to the expectation that something is wrong and that this wrongness lives within the child rather than in relationships that have been missing the child's own realities.

But here is the paradox, and perhaps the place where we can put on our hiking boots: *fix* derives from Latin "to dig; a ditch, a moat; and—to fasten." To *fasten* puts us in touch with crossing the ditch or the moat, attaching. We are then faced with a choice and a commitment from within our own selves: what might we offer these children? Will we hope to fix, or to fasten? And where will we challenge ourselves and our own struggles about uncertainty (unfastenedness) in order to make the commitment to fasten our children to their own path, a path that re-creates trust in the sense and purpose of the young self?

Logical, cognition-guided engagement with the child jeopardizes the child's own rapport with the therapist. Working with such young children demands that the therapist ensure an affect-determined presence that is trained and compassionate. Mutually affective experiences that arise are the constellations of two people who risk finding one another, and in the discovery, new forms of "fitting together" occur (Bromberg, 2011). These moments of co-exchange are a new location for both. It is the therapist's task to comprehend what has occurred and bring her understanding into the relationship. One way to do this is to introduce new affect material through the use of toys. One example is the therapist's use of narration with two puppets that can embody new insights. The puppets convey the safety of narrating feelings that the child has difficulty directly facing. The process of building the "us" is a multifaceted overlapping journey that begins with the child's desire to be known.

Process and Content

The child has been concerned, in his dependent state, that he be recognized and known as the human being that he is. With emphasis on process, a caring adult resonates with the child's meanings and perceptions so that the child can take deeper emotional risks. He relies on trusting the adult in order to practice, over and over and over, a growing interdependence in which he has something to offer. The child also depends on the trustworthy adult to give emotional feedback, which lies in the resonance between the two rather than in words. It is in this in-between gap of having something to offer that the child is motivated to sort, store, and communicate information. Through play, he has attained the stamina to think about his emotional world, where he is most vulnerable.

Trauma in Early Development

Young children have not made it to that developmental milestone of thinking about their feelings. This absence of judgment can reach into adult life when trauma has disturbed early growth. A child's reality is based on vulnerable and empathic feelings which are communicated in body language and facial expressions. We have the profound opportunity to enter directly into the perceptions of our little people, not what it felt like, but what it IS; what is now and who is feeling now. The therapist must create safety for each child's "who am I" to enter into the language of images and symbols, a speech common to all young children. Ultimately, this world of images is, in our youngest, a dreaming space, expressed naturally in metaphor and play.

The articulation of implicit memory, and then implicit reality, occurs in play and attunement. That world carries in itself strong feelings and tones, which express the tacit understanding within the child. We might say that each of us has our very own creation myth. Language is the mediator, the dynamic that encodes one's own meaning-making, files it into a subjective (me-ridden) order, and builds a history from this authorship. This is not the language of explanations and reason. A child's language is alive and stunning when we keep it in its subjective development, as the result of image-building rather than the verbal go-to resource for communication. This will hopefully assist us in crediting just how young children do communicate.

Trauma's Limbic Overdrive

There is an important possibility that occurs in young children who experience trauma. The limbic system, located deep in the base of the brain, carries our instincts and our survival. It is the ground floor imprint, providing the first connections between mother and baby. Throughout the dance of attachment, implicit memory, with its perceptions and subjectivity, is working away. The limbic system gives implicit reality something to hang onto, since the limbic brain signals when it is safe and when not. It serves as a beacon for feelings that are entering the right side of the brain, which we will discuss more in future chapters.

If the limbic system has been sending out alarms too often, the right-brain hemisphere is not given time and energy to register feelings safely. Those feelings are being recorded as "Oh oh!" and "Help!" and "Get out now!" The right hemisphere registers disturbance, and it shuts down these incoming messages in order to remain congruent with the limbic's alarms to fight, flee, or freeze.

Developmentally, the danger is that this premature filtering system will encourage a more brittle relational response. It needs to have an answer, not more feelings. The perceptive fields in the mind become undernourished when the survival brain has repeatedly set off alarms. Curiosity remains sidelined. Curiosity is the primary ingredient to imagination and future problem-solving. An effort to make sense of input that seems dangerous is shunted to the side. As we mature, we build intelligent defenses that seem justified in their establishment. Relationships hiccup along, worried and uncertain, and simultaneously call out for inclusion.

When intelligence has been needed too early in the child's life, the signals between feeling and thinking agents of the self are difficult to hear and to organize because there is a lot of static between me and what you feel about me. For instance, if the child has been in foster care twice by age five, he is not sure he is going to trust, much less hear, the signals from within that denote safe intimacy because the adults who were meant to consistently hold and mentor this position were lacking. He will more often sense something that will make him behave impulsively. The limbic system within the child is chronically alert to safety, and these alarms dictate the child's own reactivity. The child moves forward into the next stages of development with a renewed effort to make use of expanding intelligence as an even better defense weapon than what he had before. The protected-self aspects continue to be in hiding.

The child therapist enters here, in this conflict between self-protection and the urgency to relate to another safely. The therapist offers what was missed: listening concern, curiosity, and recognition of need for safe narration of the bedlam of feeling states. In a real sense, the therapist of young children interfaces with the child's perceptions of poor relationship, offering through rapport and mirroring what this child deserved from the get-go.

What can the child tell us she *knows,* in order that we might experience *our* aha moment for having discovered that particular child's knowing? Here is the link-up, the attunement itself. A mind capable of dreaming together, the natural experience of the parent's empathy, is required. Mutuality is the belief that two are together and these two states of being are in one location. A 3-year old whose work is revealed later on called this the "Usman" place. I call this co-transference: discovering together through playing together.

Unconditional open curiosity is the link-up the child requires, and having found its presence, agrees to depend on our guidance. It is the adult response to the child's intentions, not merely to his actions, which helps the child place his needs and wishes into perspective. That perspective becomes bound together, like paragraphs on a page, as the adult remains wired up and devotedly curious, waiting for the child's next inner-to-outer, images-into-ideas, and ideas-into-reflections. Control in the child remains within his range of action. Trust sustains dependency on the wired-up adult for increased comprehension of what is surfacing for understanding. The child is able to practice safely and to practice some more in figuring out empathy and the ability to self-correct when he finds himself in a corner. The worthiness that an adult offers a child will become the child's own measuring rod of self-worth. Meaning still harbors its felt-ness, its own location within the child's essential development or map-making.

Co-transference in Attunement

When I myself am not fully present, the child immediately establishes a limited presence also. Any internal conflict that may have revealed itself in the use of the toys is now battened down.

Introduction: Being Seen

The child will shield the hurt self that had begun to show itself in play, and the trauma becomes less available to be seen. It is to the degree that the therapist's self is present that the child can uncloak, become available for being seen, become known, and create change together. The unity of two establishes the third space in which both are changed.

Let me repeat this about relationship, as its import slips out of view quickly. A child, for example, is in therapy for repeated aggression at school. The therapist's first task is to be found trustworthy, emotionally safe. To the therapist, the child is not here because of aggression, but because something in this child's behavior communicates a need for understanding. As the child relaxes in the presence of this other, play increases in its intensity and in its dynamics: its order/disorder, theme repetition or not, rigidity/flexibilty, etc. Aggression enters the room, now locating itself in play. The toys might do battle with such fierceness that they are in danger of breaking. The therapist securely holds the polar tensions in the play, even while the therapist invokes curiosity toward the child's metaphors. The work with children explores this tension, revealing how each child approaches the vulnerability of being seen.

In adequate development, young children have not left, and yet are leaving, a healthy state of me-ism, of being the center of their own world and of another's whose world is intimately engaged with them. The parental sheath, this envelope of knowing what the child innocently assumes the parent is to them, is left behind gradually, as the interior empowerment of the child's self practices its strength. The meaning of *dependence* is "subordination to something needed or greatly desired" (*American Heritage Dictionary, 1992*). Dependence here is synergistic. In this intimacy the child has the trust and the safety that has been built to be able to shed this centralizing cocoon and approach the question of two importances in relationship.

Both implicit and explicit memory have been an enormous adherent to attunement, to the vulnerabilities of bonding, and to mutual recognition. They both play a part when bonding has not happened. However, within the processes of attunement and change, implicit or felt memory is the dynamic that keeps each child from being alone. The child's own internal antennae register the presence, or lack of it, in another. The more fully the child is understood and held, the more meaning is given to the mutual experience as worthy of storage. Storage is not what we did together but who we were together. Implicit memory is the record-keeper of relationship. Procedural memory might be fact-checked by others who were there or who had experiences with the same people as we did. Implicit memory is feeling-to-feeling, and fact-checking might safely follow when wanted.

When feelings are too powerful or too charged to be known in any way, a form of trance or dissociation develops and remains in place. A child's temper tantrum in many ways is the child's own efforts to discharge overwhelming feelings. The child cannot yet use narration to shift distress into the language of words, so behaviors do this task for her. In the same manner, seemingly sudden or random reactive behaviors in school may well be the only communication the child has available which, if it could be put into words, might sound something like "That kid over there just reached out and took my blocks I had for counting, and then his friend laughed at me." The teacher, having seen none of this, reprimands the child who is now overwhelmed. This silent mid-space, the space of no-words and flooded feelings, is where therapeutic relationship enters.

The implicit perceptions in the right brain are preoccupied with something truthful, something that is *me* and *mine* because of *us*. There is standing-room-only for the two people who are being vulnerable to what is next, what is here. Implicit memory is a form and a consequence of recognition. What remains alive, living, and in our memories is the shared understanding, the space where two people stand and listen and assure that meaning happens through the course of relationship.

Doing the Work

Entering the therapy session takes focus. Prior to greeting each child, I must scan myself. The child's first safety measure will be to see if I am all-here, available. She will make unconscious decisions around how much of me she finds present. Examples of distractions in me include feverishly finishing a summary of the last two sessions with other children, knowing that this child arriving is in the deep aspects of learning to trust the work and myself. Am I also wondering if I can hold the container for this child's demands? Is my drive to get reports done an unconscious determination to slow down the emotional train that's coming in 5 minutes? Instead, I need to go into the playroom. I want to open up my curiosity to what these toys will help this child say in the next hour. I bring an internal focus to knowing the integrity of this child, though I don't yet know how I will be made use of.

It is the therapist's task to bring the unnarrated story within the child's experience toward understanding, without the dependency of words in the telling. This is the task that can make therapists question their ability to work with the very young: if I cannot rely on language, how do I know that a little person and I are reaching our goals? The very fact that the story the child might reveal may have few words throws us into a world that questions our own professional belief systems: "I must know where I'm going in order to help the child get on a healing path." Not so. You must know where the child is who has survived in order to be trustworthy enough to find a new pathway through the rubble together.

When the child feels the therapist's surrendering presence in the room, the search for healing begins. The child uses the therapist's self to discover her own feeling states. If shame holds the larger state of emotional discomfort, the therapist is bound to feel shame. This mutual transference informs the conscious therapist about what needs protection from the child's own self. Co-transference *is* the relationship, and it has released the child's past harm into this presence. The feeling states are now capable of finding their representatives in the sandplay and in this intimate and professional relationship. It demands a state of reverie and openness to hold open the child's capacity to return to harmed spaces. Here is the alchemy, the transforming agent, that invokes original safety and the ability to try again. The children in this book enter that mutual space in order to restore the trust that is required for healthy relationship.

We therapists often play the part of the other in the child's story, and in the co-transference, our part overlaps that of the child's. We are given a task within the realm of the child's imagination. In this "us" space, the child's meanings are symbolized, brought into life. And in this creative adventure, the child both creates his story and sees himself in the symbol itself, perhaps for the first time. Something neither of us knew about surfaces, and we experience its newness together. The image has taken hold in the co-transference, and we are both playing in this sacred workspace.

Technique and Process

However much it might be soothing to itemize a list of "doings" or techniques, there are few in the realm of relationship. The children's stories throughout this book *are* their relationships, their dances. Their efforts to tell their stories through the toys and through relationship carry the footprints with which to approach them. The meanings are sometimes almost out of reach, almost, but not quite.

Play therapy is no free-for-all. The room has organization and structure within its setup, and the therapist is responsible for this sense of outward order. At the beginning of the hour the toys sit where they sat last week. The sand is no longer on the floor: the space invites the child in its quiet way. Quiet here means that the child can look upon the shelves and see the same dragon that expressed last week's overwhelming power. At the beginning of the hour, the child is able to ponder whether the dragon has carried the conversation far enough or if there is still more to say about the domination the dragon has conveyed. The therapist brings the memory of last week along, while not instigating its story. It is as if the therapist brings in the book with its marker of having reached chapter eight. The therapist gives the book to the child, saying, "This is your story. Where would you like to begin today?"

When the therapy relationship is in place, the toys dress in the feelings, experiences, and wishes of the child. Each session, through the movement and tension of the chosen toys, builds upon a series of themes. The changing nuances of the dramatic play unmask the child's own perceptions. The therapist remains balanced between information from the child's own home and school environments, and from the child's interior environment. The braiding of both of these contains the child's story. The change agent is the child's self.

The therapist's own interior work has stabilized into a multi-faceted orchestra of self-aspects enough so that as he joins with the child, the therapist is not lost. Techniques certainly build some bravery as we set out on the trails of finding these hurting children wherever they may be hiding from further pain. Yet, it takes ongoing awareness to keep fixing tools out of the playroom. Technique may want to keep us safe while we hope that the child, who has not been safe, will simply jump into our life raft and change feelings states. The child's genuineness demands the very human presence of the therapist's self.

So how do we go here, we who are trained to know and to use the best technique to "help" the child? This book explores when something has gone wrong. But more so, ultimately it is about righting relationship through the same trust the child requires at birth. When harm has occurred, the psyche endeavors to defend the self from annihilation by concealing it for the sake of protection within deep unconscious regions of the psyche. In this hidden place, the child suffers somatically and emotionally until the lost aspects can be safely found and re-embodied. In this, the child and the therapist enlist a third entity, the Us in the relationship, to reclaim lost aspects of psyche, or Self. Several chapters explore what "us" means to the child, with the child's expressions revealing this need for mutuality.

Part I
Between Child and Therapist

CHAPTER 1

Delilah: Not Remembering

Trust is the single-most crucial ingredient of dependency, the state of leaning into another to be understood and accepted. It is the primary and the primal aspect of the faith and expectation in someone other than ourselves that who I am will be cared for and understood. It is *through* our belief and trust in the child's wholeness that each child discovers his own lost trust in his paths. He is not looking to behave better, but rather to be *understood* better.

We approach safety as if we are referring to teaching a child to cross a busy street. In the newborn, however, safety is absolute dependency, an unconditional trust from the self that states, "Without you there is no me." The follow-up to this is "Please keep me alive." In this, safety is about intimacy. Put best, this book addresses intimate safety, the profound reliance on another human being. Relationship originates from this place of faith that someone must know what the child is doing, because this newborn "I" is in that adult's hands. And, we hope, in that adult's mind. Trust in one's self is not a given, just as trust in another is a learned experience. The therapist enters into the cracks and the static of the child's experiences that have formed each child from infancy. The beginnings of trust are located in the dynamics of claiming and cuing. In the infant, claiming provides the resonance and mirroring that the baby experiences as safety and presence. Cuing is the art of reflecting back to the infant that the parent understands this little being, and that an accurate response comes from the parent when the baby dysregulates. Cuing and claiming are requirements that provide the infant with deepening attachment. These very early dynamics are often what is missing when therapists initiate relationship with traumatized children.

Delilah, age 6, is highly intelligent and extremely sensitive. Neither she nor her parents know that about her as we begin our relationship. She shows an increasing degree of obsessions and compulsions. When we begin our work together, Delilah's panic is evident. She can hardly stay in the room with me. After two sessions, we agree that Mom will check in at the beginning of each session. In this situation it seems that Delilah carries something that she must make known to her mother. Her first images are bizarre, with animals performing positions that make no sense. They hang upside down, on top of one another, and oddly balanced on horns and hooves. I feel disoriented and without language. I have no idea if the animals are a test for me or a sensation in Delilah that reveals a mind with too much tension.

What is Delilah saying? Because the family tensions are so high, and at times Delilah's older brother is the victim of Delilah's attacks, should I jump to a diagnosis that makes us all feel less engaged with her panic? A diagnosis will provide us with names and references with behavior that needs repair. It might diminish our discomfort toward a child's interior world. It can be so appealing when we feel lost or concerned and must pull over to the side of the road because we need to check the map. Except that early in the work, we have not been given any map other than those who have gone before us. Even those maps are a bit tricky because they have not tracked this particular child. So we begin at the beginning, unsure of what Delilah's animals, in their disorganized positions, are telling us. If we work out some details about the brain in order to better understand Delilah's needs, we may be more able to know where and how to support her.

The Brain

We all know something about the brain and its workings, and we are learning more all the time. And this can be a helpful map. Maps will not tell us when we have reached our destination, what the culture will look and feel like when we arrive, or even what adjustments we may need to create when we have covered some distance. They can, however, be useful in telling us where to look in the environment when we feel a bit lost. The map we create will serve as a point of reference in learning to track children rather than as a focus on the brain's own mechanics. Maps are designs that get the traveler safely to a destination As such, brain information will help us reach the interior of a child's way of being rather than an outline of dynamics and behaviors. We will build upon it with the stories of the children themselves. Their contexts will put landmarks on our map. Their topographical markers will give us some reassurance that we are following their treasurable footprints, helping us to continue. When we are able to follow the often vague tracks in the scree, we also feel chaos and doubt whether those prints will offer up any understanding. The brain serves as a starting point in part because we have learned much about the dynamics that arise from the wirings and firings in this great organ. Before we strap on the tool belts we may need on this trek into the woods and beyond, we need to know the landscapes. Knowing the interactions in the brain provides insight and fosters compassion for each child's efforts to be understood. Our efforts to understand the child and the child's behaviors as a personal language puts us in touch with our destination: to find the child.

Current studies peer into the connections between our neurology and our less visible but powerful mind centers.

Daniel Siegel (2017), a psychiatrist who combines the science of neurology with the nature of consciousness, is one of several people writing about the mind and its mysteries. He comes from concrete research of the brain and neurology and moves about in the meaning-makers of our selves. In addition, depth psychology Jungian analysts such as Ann Belford Ulanov (2007, 2011, 2017) bring more narration to the world of dreaming, art, and healing. Neurology offers a beginning template that keeps ground under our feet as we choose to follow the small markings we are given. Ultimately, if we can comprehend that children live more deeply in their not-yet-complicated creative selves, we might have another layer with which to understand the work we offer.

Understanding the brain and its neurological structure can enable us to move more freely toward concepts of child development and what occurs in healthy relationship. Brain neurology is at the heart of what Siegel (2011, 2017) calls wiring and firing between two people. Wiring up and finding mutuality and resonance is the baby's first experience of safety. Safety creates trust. And trust is the grounding wire to healthy relationship. Some knowledge of brain "wiring and firing" points us toward relational exchanges that in turn deliver us to the inner landscapes we believe exist. We strive to track the inner workings of each child we see. A child's interior is itself the interaction of relationship. Each child creates a sense of self out of relating with another. Ultimately we track the nature of love itself, and the child's takeaway from the relationships he lives within.

The wiring that is relationship carries the full effort of the baby's development. When there is not enough access to the parent, enough wiring up for attachment to develop safely, the infant's brain remains in a constant state of dysregulation. This inability to find the parent in order to establish and maintain a sense of safety and trust overwhelms the young infant, and sets up hyperarousal that cries for connection. When we speak of poor attachment styles, we are addressing various emotional states that have resulted from excessive lack in the parent-child relationship. Because right-brain aspects create meaning prior to logic, early neglect and trauma cannot be tangibly checked for their degrees of harm. Feelings of harm must create some kind of protection, any haphazard security from further danger. These emotional states, and the neglect that created them, have no verbal language within the young child. By the time the child reaches pre-school, the brain has built reactive defenses meant to protect the child from further dysregulation and loss of safe relationship. The language we meet is the language of behaviors.

We already have examples of depth work that heals the heart of trauma in adults from authors working with this population (Ulanov, Benjamin, Kalsched). What might be available if we discuss the spirit of the child prior to and during hard-wiring of trauma before we turn to fixing the behaviors? When behaviors are not the focus of attention, they serve a more useful challenge as clues rather than outcomes. In the scenery of a child's landscape, behaviors act as the broken twigs and the overturned underbrush that point to interior decisions made by the child's self. Behaviors we hear about during intakes serve as doorways into meanings we don't yet know, which are being directed from the inside out. It will not help the child's hurts to stay on the outside of the child's welfare, correcting what the adults in their life find disturbing.

Most children have not given up the softer edges of their need to be known and their not-yet-conditioned (and conditional) ways of being in their relationships. Therefore, we adults who spend time with these children have the opportunity to find each child when his environments have cost him his trust in adults. This is the wonder and the urgency and the hope of working with the very young: the children are still counting on someone to see them. Their future emotional survival can depend on it.

After some difficulty in finding one another or wiring up into relationship, Delilah seems to sink into a harsh depression. Her breathing is slow, and she often sighs. In one early sandtray, she lays down the outer parts of certain people: their hats, armor, and skirts, with no people in them. It feels like a graveyard to me, and something more than that even; a kind of absence that has no meaning. I feel her depression and its occupancy in the disconnected parts of items without people.

Delilah is not enrolled in any school, and I strongly urge the parents to find a small program. They enroll her in a homeschool program that is willing to stay with her now constant selective mutism. Delilah is becoming more and more obsessive about visual and verbal occurrences. In the tray, she goes back to the outer fragments and shells of people and adds a casket. At one point she says out loud, "You can't tell which way to go, too covered up." The relationship between us is fragile and messy, not thoroughly conveying to me Delilah's feelings. Her feelings seem to be out of sight, unwilling to surface for me to understand. I stay with this possibility. At one point, a small miniature girl enters the wet tray. In the story Delilah is portraying, this child is the only one who can go back and forth between wet and dry. Anyone or anything else is stuck. This is Delilah's first use of a miniature who represents her self. The little girl has potential. There may be some hope here, some movement. The back and forth that this little girl initiates reminds me of the infant's need to be rocked, back and forth, helping to build trust through movement. At the same time, there is no one else seeing who she is. Delilah shows me that she herself might move from being stuck, toward trust-finding.

There is so much here, isn't there? Throughout this work we will take up the journeys of one child at a time, each blindly learning to trust the work and the relationship of being witnessed, to recover trust in themselves. This trust is the foundation of healthy relationship. To respond, and more so, to react to children's behaviors, we may unknowingly set up a choreography of doing to the child, who must then reside in being-done-to. "Doing to" takes us to fixing the child. And yet, it is *through* our belief and trust in the child's wholeness that each child discovers his own lost trust in his paths. He is not looking to behave better, but rather to be *understood* better (Benjamin, 2018).

Knowing a little about the brain helps us travel into the subtleties of relationship, whose undercurrents guide and sometimes control who we are and what we understand between one another. It is not merely the brain that makes us who we are, rather it is the interactions between the complex dynamics of the mind. Neurology demonstrates the more visible indicators of the less visible nuances of our effects on one another. Neurology strives to identify what we are doing together in our walkabouts, who is in the lead, and how the other is following; where we are and when are we just chaotically in love. We are an interconnected web of neurologies. This web is created and sustained by how we interact, how we hold one another in our own minds, thoughts, and feelings. These interactions are loosely referred to as dynamics. The primary task of therapy is in comprehending and then guiding ourselves and others within and around these dynamics. Behavior follows relationship and its dynamics, and is the result of relational connections.

All told, I worked with Delilah for about three years. I separately consulted with the parents more often than the committed monthly parent consults. Mom stayed for 10-to-15 minute check-ins during about half of Delilah's process. Mom and Dad had divorced when Delilah was four, and she and her two brothers moved back and forth between the two homes with some regularity.

Delilah's mom reports to me that Delilah's screaming at home is escalating, although she is still primarily mute in sessions. Delilah has become very anxious about going out of the house at all. Her screaming seems random. Mom can't name any reason for when this behavior occurs. I wonder internally about the dysregulation that this behavior indicates. Delilah hisses at her mom to not tell me these things, and again I model that the adults are addressing what might help to understand Delilah. She puts boats in the wet and tries to balance people in them. I "step into" her metaphor and say it is like two people in a boat, and that you need to know how to stand and not bring in water. Both Mom and Delilah chuckle. I say maybe according to Delilah a big wave is coming and according to Mom no wave is coming. So if Mom does not see the wave, maybe everyone is going to drown. Her mom tells Delilah she is so scared to give in to Delilah's extreme emotions and for Delilah, it must feel like a big wall is up between them. Delilah speaks to Mom, and says Mom lies when she knows the truth. I grab that and say it must feel like Mom is lying when she is just not sure what to say at all. Now is not the time to approach the behaviors of each of these people. I can sense that some dynamic, very old in its activity, is coming into view.

After Mom leaves, Delilah puts six adults in a bed, and a baby tucked away in a corner. The baby seems so unnoticed. Perhaps the adult world takes up so much space that this child finds herself retreating into a more obsessive world that ideally provides a sense of government and control. Nonetheless, Delilah has perhaps again created movement: a still younger self-image, gaining some landscape out of the mess of depression. Her images strike me as her own personal creation myth: the mud of beginnings and dismembered pieces slowly finding the energy to collect together. I am a bit worried as I contain the tensions between depression and screaming. I empathize with Delilah's depressive swampiness, having slip-slopped about in it as a child myself.

The Between Location

The spaces in which we find ourselves at work are within the child's meanings, and between therapist and child. This between location, if you will, is difficult to put into accurate language.

And yet it demands our efforts. Delilah was insisting that I step into this murky landscape, one without many words coming from her interior self. There was little thinking and still less mapping. I would need to trust this space. Between has few short-term measurements in a society of science that demands proof of success through the ability to measure. Measurement requires a beginning point and an end point, and goals to assist us in not feeling lost. For example, we often have a set number of sessions in which to improve the child's behaviors. To measure supports to fix, to put into unalterable form: (American Heritage Dictionary, 1992). Fixing someone may assure us that we have done all that we set out to do. On the other hand, "between" creates anxiety because there is no concrete footprint from this less visible map. The space between two people continuously refreshes itself, and thus requires an unfixed position in order to understand what is truly happening. The thin space between my skin and yours is the between space of tension that rises and falls as we trace shared understandings, and arrive for short intervals at one another's gates.

The root of *between* is *dwo*: meaning "two; at the middle point of two." It refers also to "hesitating between two alternatives" (American Heritage Dictionary, 1992). What does it mean and what does it take to remain a bit exposed ourselves, a little hesitant in order to risk finding the child's self rather than keeping to our own fixed position? Staying here for any length of time assists a child in recovering her own trust in herself and her emotions. In order to stand by at the middle point of two, our own trust needs to have been built. This is the dance of two, the *between* of relationship.

There is something between Mom and Delilah that is absent. As I hunt for what enters with the two of them each week, I attend to what I cannot hear. There is no common story between them, and Delilah seems to know this in a place inside that has no words.

Delilah tries to tell me about this loss of story in her play scenes, where the mother is far apart from the child and the child's needs. I sense her depression within myself, and let it sit in the room to help me understand. The story itself has been deleted or negated, and the further we go into its absence the more we uncover its need. This sends Delilah into severe obsessive-compulsive behaviors. At one point she becomes so distraught that the neighbors fear that abuse is happening. She begins hoarding anything that comes into the house that has words on it: envelopes, grocery lists, food labels. My attention and understanding seem to fall into oblivion, a black hole that gives me no information. My consultation group witnesses the work between Delilah and myself as I allow myself to feel around in this hole of blackness. My group is reliable: I am able to expose the sensations of my own frightening helplessness, which helps me to stay with Delilah's expanding chaos. Delilah seems to teeter between angry aggression and depression.

This is the dynamic space that reinvents itself through the experience of safe relationship. Carrying that, the maps we are given as therapists have meaning: trustworthy witnesses who understand or at least trust where we are going (supervision and consultation), the steps along the way (progress notes), our intentions (treatment plan), and knowledge that we have been here before (outcome). And supervision offers more safety for our journeying. Progress notes are crossroad markers that track the paths we choose to take, and if lost, tell us where we might pick up the trail. A treatment plan merely assures others that we are indeed tracking in the service of another. If we are able to be honest in narrating what we are finding out with this particular child, this plan will help us, too. Too often when we track the child as a whole being, the going is deep and slow. A treatment plan exposes us to the world of measurements, and how thoroughly we are tracking. We need to believe in the progress of trust in the relationship, which may not have a lot to say to others, especially in its early phases. The treatment plan is not a judge of speed, and if we remember this, using it has merit. The outcome shows us where the child's trust has taken the two of us, therapist and child. There will be markers along the way, cairns from those who have found their way into the process and have established trust. And we will signal our own markers of what and how our child clients find healing.

We therapists are called upon to understand the push and pull of dynamics and relationship in order to be available consistently as the child reaches toward that place of recovered resilience and the willingness to try again. Without this comprehension we are the blind meandering about with the blind.

Mapping Relationship in the Brain

The brain is our very simple working model that helps us approach dynamics. You might look at the brain as having four primary sections, rather than the two that are commonly defined. Some authors call out that we have five; this number depends on where we want to go with our information. We have a lot of information about the right and left hemispheres. There is also a frontal lobe manager and a more primitive reptilian back seat driver to the brain, called the limbic system. The frontal lobe is the oversight executive function. The limbic system, in the rear central of the cranium, carries the job of instincts and survival. It speaks most quickly to the body in its use of our senses. The limbic system is the original construct which keeps us tied to our more primitive needs of safety and survival. This part of the brain, the fight-flight-freeze center, oversees the body and its responses to input. Loosely put, the limbic system has a lot of management over our behaviors and our impulse control. The limbic system serves both the left and right hemispheres of the brain, and its demands will gradually be incorporated into more mature intracommunication. In the very young infant, we might imagine that this system is sending telegraphic messages to the baby's neurosystem, whose messages are creating a body. This body, when sufficiently informed, separates the baby from the mother's self, and sets up a home, you might say, in that baby's body. The body establishes the growing withdrawal from what has been the baby's mutuality of *us*.

The structure of the brain holds the first entries into the work of our children. The three primary neurological dynamics build their way toward smooth interaction within the very young child. The right hemisphere will build the stamina to observe a feeling and create a perspective. It makes sense of our non-verbal signals such as facial expression, tone of voice, gestures, while the left side is taken up with cause and effect. The right hemisphere is ready to go at birth. Its first primary information is sensate and holistic. Many of its capacities develop in a gathering sort of fashion, learning and storing competencies that will activate in increasingly complex manners after age three. The left hemisphere is engaged in reasoning, logic, and the use of language to communicate. Left-brain dynamics will make constant adjustments to calm impulsivity and turn it toward thinking. However, its beginnings, of being held by the governing care of a receptive adult, hold the keys to future interaction of these brain and mind dynamics.

Activity between front, sides, and rear brain systems creates a series of subtle adjustments in the brain and throughout our bodies, as both our interior and exterior environments respond to stimuli, intuit safety, make meanings, and then modify meanings according to how confidently we experience ourselves in relationship to others. As the more sophisticated areas of the brain mature, they will govern over the more primitive aspects. I will discuss these brain managers further in context to relationship and behavior. Because the attention in this book is on very young children, we will focus most heavily on the relationship between the limbic and right-brain systems, the two fields in the brain that carry the young child's meanings most deeply and yet very nonverbally.

How does the baby inaugurate a "me" that is separated from the "us" of the mother/baby symbiosis? The limbic system actually holds many of the secrets of embodiment, of not merely taking it for granted that we *have* bodies, but that these bodies allow us to safely separate and become a self. Embodiment must have enough trust and love of another to allow this separation, this stepping onto the dance floor and giving in to the persistent interaction of self and other, other and self.

Delilah works hard to show me what she knows and cannot put into verbal language. In her efforts to reveal her feelings, Delilah again uses a family who fall from the boat. They are all covered with sand. Delilah forces sand into their mouths. Not only are they drowning, they are also speechless regarding their experiences. I am slowly getting it. In my concern, I insist on a psychological evaluation, all the while feeling intuitively that this inquiry is for me and not for Delilah. Slowly, Delilah listens to me talking with Mom about the stories her child needs to hear, stories of Mom's childhood and of her daughter's birth and of their experiences together. Obsessions lessen. The words that had been piling up in Delilah's room, letters and grocery lists and reminders, taper off a little.

I find out that Mom has no story of her own birth. She herself was adopted and she has no memory of her childhood. She has no stamina to find out what her history is; it is simply too overwhelming. This overwhelm may be the drowning and the voicelessness that these two highly sensitive people share. A bit later on, I find out the dad was adopted, also. The two may be struggling for enough fastening between one another, leaving Delilah too unattached, or too attached to their own untold stories. An added probability is that Delilah's older brother has found enough room in his parents' lives to have experienced attachment, which makes Delilah a bit more obviously the identified problem.

Vigilance

Right-brain vigilance can help us understand some of the unwanted behaviors of children in schools. These behaviors are a result of neurological pathways that have been laid down to protect the child from feeling engulfed by others' feeling states. These pathways are affected by external overwhelm, subtle combinations of temperament, levels of intelligence, and other influences. There is no black and white category that can separate nature from nurture. In fact, past a certain point there is little reason to separate these sophisticated concepts. As our brains develop, with cells firing and therefore creating us moment by moment, we braid internal and external experience that is always in the process of being and becoming who we are. The right brain also carries the capacity for a depth that can be experienced as transpersonal.

In states of intense pressures and survival, defenses will paradoxically take care of us until a trigger is hit. Self-protection guards against potential danger. It rests in the space between two, where parental curiosity, focus, and claiming isn't strong enough. The real danger has already occurred, and the effort to keep that from being felt again remains in place. The internal demand for relief results in unbearable behaviors. Enough trust must be built so that the child wants relief from intolerable feelings, even risking feelings from the danger yet again. Who of us in a child's world will tolerate these outbreaks of feelings enough, in order to relieve the child through core wiring of compassion, reflection, and empathy? Our trustworthy presence will ignite the child's urgency to be seen again. The child will confront a tipping point of a dilemma: to remain protected and defended or to risk the potential of trust. When trust approaches, this conflict between remaining defended and finding relief shows up as chaos. This must be addressed: one part of the child is reaching for attachment and another part increases its vigilance and hostility or invisibility, with the goal that past danger not appear again.

One job of therapists, teachers, and parents is to give space and attention to the many, many nuances within a child's neurology: the alerts when attachment is threatened, the relaxation when the child feels understood and, more than that, is allowed to remain in what is happening while the adult nurtures that child toward renewed security. The hints and smatterings from the child's interiors are those notes that were molded into the neurological construction. They are about "me" before "I" had any choice. They are not about the child; they *are* the child. And as the child approaches the longing to grab a waiting hand there may likely be an increase in impulsive and compulsive behaviors. We will likely see the internal dilemma of stay away and come closer manifesting in chaotic dysrhythmic intensities.

The "me before I chose a me" is the child's experience. Because the brain is not yet mature or experienced in a solid-enough self, she constantly reaches for the containing adult who will mentor her toward this solidification. Each time the child finds an adult safely reaching toward her, the child's own neurology builds a little more confidence, a little more satisfaction in finding separation. It cannot be emphasized enough: the child's sense of self depends on the relationship that she is wired up to. She receives the information of who she is in this current between two people.

Delilah's anxiety has reached the level of attacks on Mom when neither of them can articulate what needs a voice. This becomes our focus, while Delilah continues to express her depression and loss of voice in tray images. Then, while a volcano enters the play and Delilah verbalizes that no one can cross the mountain because of the fear of explosions, she also starts making some stories. She quietly mutters their content to her mother, while I listen in. Her attacks stop suddenly when Delilah begins physically shadowing her parents everywhere. She cannot let them out of her sight. Both parents report that they feel their daughter is more connected, although they are very tired from her demands. I ponder how Delilah is bringing newness to her relationship with her parents. She is no longer giving in to a no-voice, no-story self. Her high beams are on so that they can find her. While she tracks them, she demands that they remember everything, including road signs that they pass on the street. She wants to know the details of being born, over and over, of all three of the children. She becomes hysterical if they forget or change story details. When I ask her about this, she is able to say to me, while facing her mom, "I'm afraid of being wrong." She wonders if she might be lying. Again, here is more context to the absence that had ruled, more meaning to this young girl's need for something that had not occurred when she was an infant.

As we move toward a benefit-of-the-doubt position and away from correcting the child's pulsing neurology, we are dancing with the child in her own perceptions and sensations. Those perceptions are the meaning making that has been attributed to the child's experiences which, when witnessed safely, are expressed in stories and self-made understandings. This is a core requirement: to make sense. When a child can move in tandem with an adult and with that adult's safety, he will internalize organizing and making sense through what the relationship emotionally contains. In this dance, the child will learn to trust our lead in slowing the dance steps of impulsivity down while not diminishing any of the child's viewpoints and markers. As the child slows a bit, he moves away from the reptilian brain toward connection with an other, and then reliance on this other. The outside, separated from the inside, becomes trustworthy. Children are determined to make sense from the inside out, which puts adults and our needs for facts and information a bit secondary!

In the playroom, Delilah is articulating more of her subjective meanings, saying them instead of acting them out. She also makes use of the toys more and more, as they carry the perceptions of her own realities into the tray. She tells Mom, "Nobody will believe me. I'll remember something you won't remember. That's crazy." In another session, she states, "You even keep forgetting what I say is the problem! See? You forget!!"

Delilah has a psychological evaluation. This helps the parents to see that how she describes her internal states has merit, while offering them some additional guidance in OCD behaviors. Delilah settles into this awareness a bit, like a baby whose parents have taken her need for a certain blanket seriously. She comments that with so many words everywhere, "Nobody outside me will remember." Here is each child's vital question: "Will you remember me?" This tells her mom the origin of Delilah's obsessions with words on envelopes and in stores. Truly nonverbal narration has been absent. Nonverbal stories are laid down before the age of one, when the parent is cuing and claiming the baby within the unique languages of the body and of comfort. Something in this patterning had not been strong enough for the baby Delilah. In the therapy room, she is attempting to coax her mom into filling in the absence of a very young self. As this child pushes herself on with verbal narration, and with physically learning to bicycle and to roller-skate, her parents hold back in their confidence of Delilah's efforts. I can see the formation of "the identified patient," and turn more attention on the parents themselves, pushing them to take on new skills on behalf of this highly sensitive child of theirs. We focus on the construction of an emotional language that the family will use together. This is a challenging step for them, as I learn that they have used their own forms of acting out rather than speech in their own relationship.

We are in a rehearsal of sorts, a rehearsal for a future that will be internally confident in its dance steps. But there is no sudden learning. That repetitive step-dance learning while fact-checking through dialogue is one central task of childhood. And the task of important adults in each child's life is to assist in this practice. It is not merely to correct those steps or to prevent them from going astray, but rather to guide the child toward and through healthy relational understanding of connection and empathy. This timeless dance offers the child an ever-expanding curiosity that builds from the child's own meanings.

Movement is from the interior to the environment. There is no developmentally specific time when the child's reasoning steps onto the stage. Rather, it is as though the right brain stretches toward the left brain, slowly and surely creating a bridge from the child's own meaning-maker, until a fundamental and authentic relationship establishes within the child's own self. The caring and attuned adult hears the child's perceptions of the world and how it works with curiosity more than needing to teach the child facts. With this rapport in place, it is a matter of time and confidence for the child to become a world traveler, if not outwardly, at least within the nearly infinite questions that erupt between imagination and fact, between feeling and doing, between image and task, ultimately, between one's own myth and one's own reality.

Importantly, when a caring and wired-up adult guides more than corrects in these interactions, the child learns flexibility. As a consequence of an attending adult, the child's neurology becomes comfortable with being empathetic over time. Relational elasticity is also the basis for curiosity about our own feelings and those of others. I need not prove I am right, since the other has listened and understood often enough. We are still making sense together. This making sense has resonance, relating together across a mutually active space.

Delilah: Not Remembering

Delilah enters the room as a trickster, crouched, with her finger shushing over her mouth, grinning. We both laugh. She's "sneaking up" on me. She announces, "You are different from yourself." I reflect this back. She uncloaks her own meaning. "Yes. 'You' has three letters; 'yourself' has eight. That makes 'you' different." This exposes the duality of her working mind: she is both tracking meaning and letters-as-meaning. Delilah had tracked the way letters go together, and perhaps this had been a soother to her persistently present anxiety. As her anxiety went beyond her thresholds of letter-tracking as a method of calming herself, the letters in the environment became the objects of her own overwhelming anxieties.

The acceptance of her intelligence and of how she has used that intelligence is more crucial than the name of the dynamic. Delilah's comprehension finally lets me understand that her early compulsive urgency about names, spellings, and creating and keeping hundreds of lists of tasks, expectations, and conversations was a clever and overwhelming effort to gain control over all those intelligent monologues within. These monologues had not enough check-points; they continued to fall into a dark hole because the words, paragraphs, and stories that might connect them were absent. Her soothing tools may have become her own enemies, devolving into the chaotic hoarding of letters of the alphabet in her room. Delilah's own remembering and being remembered was triggered to the point of disabling her.

Left-Brain Development

Children are born with both right and left-brain hemispheres, but they are right-brain dominant through most of childhood. Development of language sharply increases left-brain growth. There is another more intense development in the left brain in adolescence. Generally, however, left-brain development is a gradual process that occurs throughout childhood (Janina Fisher, 2017). Imagine how much practicing, updating, and yet more practicing is required of the growing governor in each child. Too often what we learn about child development outlines the left side of the brain, leaving the right side of the brain mysterious and unheard from. And yet, as play therapists, we are working with the firings of the right brain. We are inter-firing. We ourselves engage in the child's past experiences of unformulated feeling-states that wired themselves into the child's ongoing perceptions and responses. Those experiences, for the child, enter this here-and-now relationship, and they test the ground between us to see if we are strong enough to stay, to wait it out, to reveal, to understand. Inter-firing is crucial. It applies to our work as therapists with young children insofar as our conscientious focus is on perception and intention as the important focus rather than more logical causes of behaviors.

One aspect of disturbance in the child's neurology is the porous filter that the child chooses, survival over attachment. Too often too much distress creates a toxic brain environment. The brain firing works to resolve this chronic disruption of the child's need for trust and initiates a greater dependency on the limbic system. The protective and the more vulnerable result here is that children's brains are highly capable of bringing survival instincts more immediately into action. Their dependency is a profound action, a verb, which we are called upon to share in as therapists when we are safe enough participants. We can throw diagnostic terms at this understanding, or we can be amazed that a child's self has its own delicate balances that, when sensing danger, allows its more primitive brain to take over. Somewhere in Delilah's very early history, she had felt forgotten. Her accusation of parental lies, and of "You don't remember!" constantly demonstrated her need for a personal, subjective story that was mirrored in her parents' felt responses to her. Her work continuously focused on her requirement to be remembered, to fill in a landscape that for her was absent of a core attachment design. Delilah's emotional sensitivities to her parents' emotions left her without mooring.

Limbic System as the Third Brain

The limbic system is immediate in its reactions, not waiting for an adult to make decisions. Trust and inter-reliability are abandoned in favor of "I trust me," this me being an inexperienced and therefore very vulnerable self. The survival brain, which moves into full operation within a 15-second window, is just this: a young brain that learns that it is safer to go it more or less alone than to rely on a connection between self and adult guide. The increased dependence on the limbic system in the brain means that the child's development is hindered by a great need for safety. Development slows down, and learning is downgraded to a crawl. Whenever the limbic system is in charge, developmental windows close down. It is the same thing we do when there is a great storm coming. We close down computers, heaters. We shutter our windows. We do what we must in order that the storm leaves minimal damage. This is what the limbic system does on behalf of the child's best interests.

There is a paradox in this state of affairs. Because the developing brain is so pliable, it calls upon areas of the brain as needed. In healthy development, the stronger and more reliable the thinking brain becomes, the more likely it is that we will learn to think about what is occurring before we react. That is referred to as impulse-control. At least that is the reigning expectation. However, a child's thought-making brain is not stable, and is not even activated for the first 5-to-8 years. The very system that supports attachment through its openness also immediately moves to separate rather than attach, without registering the consequences. If the child feels overwhelmed, not safe, or frightened, the limbic system, that survival part of the brain, steps in. The paradox is that children have a knee-jerk access to defending themselves, a requirement, for children so dependent on their environments and not able to choose their surroundings. In a real sense, adults *are* the environment; they are the lead in the dance.

Recall that Delilah was able to tell her mother that Mom told lies. This overarching statement was a narration that made it to the surface after 6 years of being solely in the parental environment. Later on, we would uncover work that was Mom's own childhood trauma. Mom's lack of attachment had created profound forgetting, leaving vacated areas that Delilah could not fill in, no matter how many letters and definitions she collected. Simultaneously, Delilah's parents had divorced as Delilah herself stretched toward some future capacity to enter school and tolerate periods of carrying strong enough parent images internally. Mom was the primary caregiver, yet Dad had also experienced an abandoned past. Individual consultations with Mom revealed very painful and poorly mirrored backgrounds for both of Delilah's parents. As Mom began her own work, Delilah's compulsions slowly lessened, revealing a little girl with tremendous levels of sensitivity and few skills with which to name herself. Vulnerability in the parent-child relationship left skill building too limited. This dynamic Delilah identified as a "lie." She had not developed a strong enough center of self, a pulsing radar that, if we roam too far, calls us back. Delilah had roamed somewhere and gotten lost, and with her mom's lost stories, Delilah felt too little when she hunted for connection. It was not that Mom did not love this child. She truly did. The lack of center and its self-confidence mirrored an absence to her daughter.

Dependency

Adults are the pathfinders for the children they hold in their minds, which lets these children know someone is tracking them and remembering them. Knowing this, we have more access to available healing within them because of this ongoing elasticity of the brain, and of the dependency that lives in children. Dependency leans deeply into the lives of others who they count on and love. Delilah was reaching out to trust and depend on her mother. With that stretch, she could continue growing emotionally. The absences were being filled in. Delilah perceived that her mom could think about her even when Delilah herself wasn't there to remind Mom of her presence and her need. This developmental phase, of trusting that the parent is present even when she's absent, is one of the critical learning acquisitions like the peek-a-boo game of a 1-year-old.

Delilah points out that she can't fit in the baby crib anymore:

Delilah tells me, as we begin to emerge together from such deep work, that the baby in the play has to give up her crib. "She doesn't want to, but she can't fit." Meanwhile, she and her mom agree that she can recreate her entire bedroom. She shows me in a drawing how she is rearranging her furniture. Her big brother can actually enjoy spending time with this little girl now, and he remarks to his parents that his sister is much smarter than most of his friends.

Delilah is growing developmentally. This quickened growth requires a ritual, and Delilah creates it herself. Her entire room reflects this interior change through an exterior re-make.

To understand the dynamics at play, we might place dependency in the broader lap of attachment. Delilah had chosen to be *un-dependent*. She had not found the link up, the place in which to find refuge often enough, as an infant. Her own risk in stretching out toward others was compromised. Dependency forges our intrinsic capacity to relate, to stand with some vulnerability and to be available to interpenetrations with others, to risk negotiating from our own truths toward the truths of the other without diminishing ourselves. Often in Delilah's sessions, I could hear her fear of being able to trust the interchange of two people. I believe that was one meaning of her assertion of mom "lying." That back-and-forth exchange that we come to rely on in healthy relationships was not nearly strong enough.

Dependency establishes our internal working models of relationship. In order to refresh this profound word that place-holds who we are in relationship to one another, let's really look into its meanings and contexts. To depend on: "to place trust or confidence [in]"; "a subordination to something needed or greatly desired"; "the state of being determined, influenced, or controlled by something [someone] else." In its root meaning, dependence derives from the Germanic derivative "the spinner, to spin" (American Heritage Dictionary, 1992). To spin: when we are interdependent, we are spinning something that neither one of us could have created in isolation. Will this effort stretch our understanding of one alone to a creative twoness that binds us more intimately? And is this what we might imply when we assume that children are influenced by someone else? Children may be said to be in "subordination to something needed or greatly desired": we are that greatly needed and greatly desired something/one.

Attachment includes dependency, and is the broader system in which dependency is embedded. It was as if Delilah had scooted her little self right into place within the family dynamics, and found relief and connection. To do so, she had had to direct her energies toward a much younger self, one that took the risks of a much stronger attachment than she had been able to build in infancy. To attach is to "connect" to "affix or append; add" (American Heritage Dictionary, 1992). Append and depend come from the same root, letting us know how closely these words travel with one another. Attachment is to "bind one thing [person] to another," to bond. Perhaps we can regain the excitement of that which we are truly tracking here, not merely an academic string of sentences that induce us into thinking, but more importantly, a root system that begs us to remember what we mean. To truly walk about inside of the larger system of attachment, therapists and parents need first to break in and establish our own map of the many subtle dimensions of what we mean by attachment. Without this initial effort, words might hide us from our own struggles to understand children and attachment through the intellectualizing our work. When this happens, we too have a metaphoric room full of empty words that pretend to tell us about ourselves.

Delilah has been learning to trust the meaning of her own words, and the narrating memory (remembering and being remembered) through the revealing of her own private stories. It comes time to test my remembering capacities: do I know this child? Will I remember her stories? Can I mirror a good enough relationship? In the tray, she sets up a map. The sand, she states, is "the human world."

"Let's go into the human world. There are five keys. They each go to a different lock which a bird protects." My first task is to remember which keys go to which locks. I remember one door to one key. "That's the key to the bird museum. The birds each have a story to tell. They whisper…" I choose the eagle. "He'll try to remember his story. He finally remembers his story. It's about living in a person's house. There's a baby crib. There's a rug. There's a plant in there. Back then he was a small, tiny bird and he slept in the baby's room. There was a T.V. that played videos so the baby would feel safe."

"They called her Baby. She was a very sensitive baby. I'm going to ask you questions, and you'll remember!" She goes on to tell me a wonderful story, with fragments of her own growth tucked in. In fact, the bird museum, with its locks and keys, may be Delilah's story of origin, or myth.

Then she asks me test questions. Her testy questions have an element of aggression in them, and my own anxiety shows itself to me, as I wonder if I will "forget." My anxiety rears up. I narrate this: "What if I forget!" I am so afraid of not remembering correctly, of "lying" when I just might not know. But, we keep going. I steady myself to be real, just simply real. I hope that Delilah's trust in me will forgive the mistakes I may make when I respond to her tests. She is now keeping a relationship connected. There is little absence of anything between us, with both of us inventing this moment in the bird museum together. She has elements of control, but is not out of control. In the final scene, the family house is orderly. The parents are together, the daughter's room has a number of articles in it: flowers, a birthday cake, books. She includes her older brother's space, which had seemed to compete with her needs early on. Now she grants him his own place in the family, one which is not threatening to her own attachments to their parents. Along with the sand images, Delilah draws a picture of a baby and a set of blocks with letters on each side of each block. Obsessive/compulsive letters have found a useful place which can construct whole towers and citadels of story. A celebration is going to happen.

As Delilah acted upon her trust in a relationship that shared mutual creativity, with no one person in control, it ceased to matter if I answered her questions rightly. What mattered was that I tried, that I showed intent curiosity and that the two of us could follow her story together. In these last sessions, it felt like our two heads were watching the same tracks in the sand, and wondering together about what we saw. Delilah had dropped her obsessions about being right or, given enough letters, she could cut and paste a story she could not feel between herself and her parents. Together, we had "tried to remember" her story, playing in the human world. And then, we had "finally remembered" and could pass on through the old vacant spaces with some letters and words, gathering in a whole story of Delilah's experiences. The full story adhered her meaning-memory with her language-memory. Her intelligence was now freed from employing letters and words which had seemed to hold her dilemma of knowing and not speaking. Her imaginative language, and the common language of children, was the language of symbol and story, the as-if language. She had recovered this original story-making world, which protected her dependent core from direct and literal confrontations. Delilah's bird museum was now an interior place we had built together, with Delilah as author and me as witness. Her own story was nested in the eagle's story. Delilah left it up to me to straddle the gap between a potential safety in language and our more discovery-oriented course. Finally, Delilah pressed herself to learn how to ride her bike and how to roller-skate. She pushed her parents to trust her to go a bit farther in physical distance than they felt ready for, stretching them to take on this newness she felt. These innovative physical challenges brought new authority and embodiment to Delilah's empowerment.

This child was ready to leave therapy, but not before telling me how frightening it had been to come see me in the beginning. It seemed important that she return to our relationship beginnings. She could remember her feelings, and could pass on to me a narrative that made complete sense to both of us. I heard after her closure that she had become a leader in her class, leaning on her intelligence to make friends. I learned more recently that she has been accepted in universities with her focus on social history and writing. Because of her intelligence, staying in university settings has been very difficult for her. She has made several time-outs at home, where she can withdraw from the over-stimulating world before taking flight again.

CHAPTER 2

Annie and the Wolf: Remembering and Memory

"There is more to remembering than neural systems. I think that if we are really to unpack the mysteries of memory, we need to put the story back into the science" (Fernyhough, 2012).

There are a multitude of influences which braid together to create our selves. In using children's own stories, we might see more clearly what they are willing to trust us with and how they teach us. We might, for instance, identify sensory integration issues or oppositional defiance: What is behind these behaviors? How much does temperament or intelligence contribute? Or, attention deficit. What do we want to understand? What are the children's own stories and experiences behind these more objective words? The work experiences of the children here are meant to reveal the necessity of being understood and being remembered. In essence, a good deal of our job description as play therapists is to find where our young clients are waiting to be found. We wait for the context of the child's experiences, through the stories the child will create from inside.

There is little immediate purpose to a diagnosis other than to provide a common use of terms so that we adults might speak to one another in more explicit language, shortening the time it takes to communicate. As we utilize efficiency, our results may shorten the distance between two people while also decreasing our capacity to resonate together and find understanding. Shorter is often, in this regard, not better. Brevity for the sake of efficiency can easily train us to lean into more objective assessments, speaking *about* the child from a series of already defined behaviors. A diagnosis will not shorten the time it takes to find the child and, having found where they hang out, to guide them toward their own hungry need to be cared for and deserving of care. To walk around in their world, let's augment what we mean by relationship by adding implicit memory, somatic memory, and being carried about in someone's mind. We who are trained to witness children carry an especially delicate responsibility. We are also asking of ourselves to understand a minority population from which we ourselves often carry bruises and scars. Understanding the implicit world of the child takes energy and curiosity.

Implicit and Explicit Memory

Implicit memory is at work in story and healing, built from felt, relationship-based understandings. These understandings consist of perceptions, feeling states, bodily sensations; and they may well show up as behaviors that no one can quite make sense of. What is implicit is not readily apparent. What meanings a 6-year-old child may have made of an experience, such as being bullied on the playground, are the consequences of all previous 6 years of how she has been understood. If she has been discounted, this bully is an outer human being of an interior experience, and she will react with the behaviors she has built-in for protection. Adults may not know, then, why she runs away near hysterics when the situation itself has no appearance of being that dramatic. Triggers from within intrinsic memory ignite that child's perceptions of harm, and activate the limbic system. Explicit memory, on the other hand, has evidence. Two children might agree that they both ran for the slide, and can debate who got there first.

Early experiences collect in feelings and perceptions. There is no repression because repression depends on the hippocampus, necessary for explicit memory, which is not mature in infancy. It's the amygdala that promotes the organization of implicit memory, and remains rich in feelings and tones. This personal history exists in each of us and plays out in our own experiences of smells, tastes, what we love and don't love. Sometimes we cannot understand why we are suddenly angry or scared while there's nothing in our presence that needs this reactive state. Implicit memory is the backbone of what we call regulation, and perhaps to go further, we can say it's the backbone of our trust in others. Having said that, it's also the reverse: the backbone to mistrust that hasn't been explicitly expressed.

Intermittent attachment is undependable for the infant. What ends up wired into the brain's neurology, the child's own touchstone of familiarity, is this unpredictability. At some point later on, even too much routine can feel foreign and unsafe. Young children in the foster care system often exhibit the unpredictability of their first caregivers by seemingly random behaviors that are actually internally wired-in maps of their own experiences. As predictability occurs, such as regular bedtimes and family meals, these little ones show sharp increases in anxiety. A neurosystem that has been built on unpredictability leans heavily into the limbic system for its dependability. The limbic system, remember, carries the speedier reactive states meant for survival. If it no longer feels safe, it demands a getaway. Or it acts up so that at the very least there is a smokescreen that will not reckon with the onrush of feelings. Adults may wonder why food is being hidden when in fact now children have easy access to good food. Or, the child is reprimanded and suddenly bites the adult. We might consider this interior survival system as an internal check-point, a self-created fantasy parent of sorts. The child will count on this fantasy parent, an impulse-ridden caretaker who is at best the child's own developmental age, and may well be much younger than the child.

Children depend on the limbic system's responses when healthy relationships aren't available to them. Therefore, the core self hasn't built an external frame of reference that serves as a growing internal resource. The two primary resources here are an external guidance that has not been a stable regulator for the young child and the ongoing internal hunger to locate an other who might bring calm to the child's great over-stimulating challenges. This emotional urgency is dumbed down gradually as the child learns that attachment creates danger. And a state of calm is vital to the capacity to organize thoughts and feelings as we grow. If we are in a state of feeling, we can't think. We who interface with children in classrooms have many examples of what occurs when implicit memory takes over. Even though a child may now be safely adopted, people coming too close physically still get attacked. Nothing in the child's current environment has set off aggression. It is the child's internal environment that reacts. We will unpack pieces of this in children's work as we look closer at attachment and implicit memory. We will look into these governing forces at work with regard to the building of esteem, its role in impulsivity, and the overall interactions of attachment and self.

Therapeutic Helplessness

The children who help us learn how to stay with them, at times in very troubled and neglected environments, have courage beyond measure. Oftentimes because we strive to keep our children safe, when we sit with a child who has not been safe and whose stories are difficult and sometimes beyond our own experiences of hurt, our reaction is to save, to overcome the hurt in front of us. As our tools of salvation become more and more meaningless in this effort, we may want to move to fixing behaviors. Helplessness is a profoundly uneasy visitor in the play-therapy room. At the very same time, allowing the helpless and hopeless into the room may make the difference to the child's sense of being seen. If adults find these feelings intolerable, the child perceives himself as intolerable, increasing those ominous feelings. The child's self is still too open to separate sensations from identity. These large dark feelings are the monsters that sit on the chests of our hurt children, devouring good feelings and creating shame. Someone needs to know of their presence, and that is one crucial job description within the title of play therapist.

Annie was 5 years old and in foster care when I saw her. Her infant brother had died from the severe neglect all the children had experienced by the birth mother and father.

In Annie's first session, she tells me, "I remember all of it, even since I was a baby." I wonder at the time if Annie is telling me that she remembers what had happened in a black-and-white sort of way. There seems to be little affect to Annie's message to me. And there are no intimate others left in Annie's life, at her very young age of five. Her social worker brings her because Annie is a ward of the state. Her siblings had been adopted; Annie alone stands in the unwanted space of waiting for a family. She knows that the family she is with will not fulfill that urgent requirement. Annie has already been in three foster placement homes because of her aggressiveness.

In the first two sessions, Annie identifies an image for her danger and how she makes use of that danger. "I got a wolf by me all the time. If there's any problem, that wolf takes care of it." And Annie is having huge difficulties with her own "wolfishness," her belief that she herself will keep out the harm she had known. With her sisters and brothers in permanent homes, and her baby brother deceased because neglect had been that profound, Annie keeps to her wolf. In short, Annie has no one to remember her.

She says her wolf is a guardian, who she sends out ahead of her. She tells me that he can lead her into Hell to find the person who hurt her brother. Later on, she moves a wolf to live under the dollhouse. I am to do nothing to help him inside. The wolf becomes both the guardian and the darkness. The wolf is also concrete in Annie's feelings. She is clear that no one is going to get through her instinctual protection; no one can hurt her like she has been hurt. This wolf brings understanding as to why Annie has already been moved to three previous foster homes. She cannot tolerate being told how to behave while listening for someone to understand her wolfishness. In this regard, she states the exact truth: "The wolf takes care of any problem."

So we start by calling that wolf in by way of its image. I bring a very detailed photo of a gray wolf, and Annie is ecstatic. She is able to give me more information about this resilient effort on her part to keep danger out. It has taken immense effort for this young child to remember herself. Her memory, as such, is an unsettled bundle of intense feelings that are laced with chronic infant loss and trauma. She is not only telling us about her brother and that loss, but also about herself and how close that disappearing is for her deeper self.

The wolf, invited in, becomes the force that has kept track of her until she can reach out to me. When she does, she is overwhelmed with feeling, some of which she lets me know we wouldn't talk about. I create rituals and routines that are simple and are fully intended to show Annie that I remember her from week to week. Because I know Annie has experienced hunger at both physical and at much deeper psychic levels, I have food ready. The food is often hard and crunchy, like apple slices, to help her include the presence of her body in this hour. I begin each hour of work with a very simple summary of what myself, Annie, and the wolf have done the previous week. I make use of simple images that she has used most recently, as if I am calling her to join me in a new kind of relationship that will be safe, if she can bear safety. She is so surprised when I can tell her the story she had built in the previous week. Her surprise seems to point at hearing an outside person—outside of her wolf barriers—thinking of her.

Fantasy as a Defense

When a child has experienced too little wiring-up as an infant, fantasy replaces relationship and attunement in the service of substitute soothing, but false organization, of self. A dissociated memory is about "me" recalling "me." This "me" is the halfheartedly-attached self attaching to something "I" fantasize into place. The wolf carried the innate place holder of care within Annie. As such, her wolf was rigidly organized. He knew just what he was needed for. Oftentimes I felt the presence of Annie's wolf as the guardian between us.

One crucial place where play heals is in the realm of memory. To risk losing fantasies of who caregivers could be in lieu of the real persons who the child really knows is profound. In play, fantasy slowly moves from its unquiet silence into a moving image, and this image balances itself in the between world of therapist and child. Once in this "in-between" space, images can begin to move, to enliven rather than freeze the feelings and needs of relationship. The images gradually become a story, and little by little interior organization takes hold. The story, revealed in play and tested on the therapist, sort of warms up. As that occurs, the child nervously learns to depend upon our own steady presence. We can say that what has been frozen begins to move about, to risk having feelings, and to risk the longings that a "you" might understand a "me." In Annie's play, the wolf was beginning to shift. His tasks in the play were moving from a low growling presence toward me, to his location at the doorway to the house. And then, he moved to guard the baby in the crib. Implicit memory was located in image now. When movement of the image played out, Annie gave me the opportunity to peer into her past without any intrusion of questions or fact-finding.

The child's memories which have been too much to bear are bearable in this space. The child accedes to trust, and in this trust, a story that knits together broken pieces of a past can be seen, heard, and made sense of. Will that story be about her losses? Not directly, but certainly the adult sharing this in-between space will feel the deep survival, fear, isolation and other feeling states that the child has experienced. Learning about Annie's wolf wasn't a comforting or comfortable place. I was often very tired as I approached Tuesday afternoon. It was as if my feet were dragging, admitting my resistance to sharing Annie's burdens and her responding wildness. I needed to set my awareness directly on and into Annie. She demanded that, and she deserved it.

During one particular session, she silently works through the hour to structure a way to hang the angel over her sand tray. The wolf is under the house, the angel over it. This image recognizes her experiences and reassures her. I feel the presence of something much bigger than either of us alone. She jumps up after I hang the angel where she instructs me to, and she yells out, "I hope God's watching all this! I hope my brother is dancing up there like crazy! I bet he's coming down here laughing his butt off! I'll never forget this, all my life. <u>You'll</u> never forget this even when you're 101 years old! Cuz once I pestered Ellen's cat, and he swiped me, and now he always swipes me, cuz I pestered him, and he never forgets me!" Annie had pestered both of us enough to begin the risk of trusting a new relationship.

This session is a turning point in Annie's trust. She moves toward me with her feelings and expresses anger. She creates clay parents and then hammers them down to flatness. She draws a large hammer with a red hammerhead. Below where it might strike she writes her birth mother's name, then dares me to say anything.

Annie and the Wolf: Remembering and Memory

"We won't talk about that, at all," she says. Anger bristles in the room as I say that talking about that is way too sad and mad right now.

I became the memory and the moderator of the play. Through a responsive attunement, I became charged with calming over-activity and bringing in the power of feeling when under-activity occurred. We can refer to this as building a new self together with a child, that includes its various feelings. The two of us ruggedly kept Annie's feelings more constantly out of her overwhelm threshold while housing the gradual energies that she could communicate. The self-states were initially states we shared, infant-like and fragile. We were traveling back through Annie's neurosystem, through implicit memories that had been stored without connections to the soothing presence of an adult.

We were building a weblike construct from within the child's own self, revealing the face of the child's own uniqueness. Together, the child and the therapist unmask the internal reality of the child and then organize reality so that child can use what is being rebuilt as a felt frame of reference. Perhaps this organizing taps into what we call memories and sort of "straightens them out" from a disarray of feelings. More internal organization occurs, and out of this organization meaning emerges. Annie's memories were risking some attention, and that attentiveness by both of us, pestering away, was beginning to loosen the black-and-white rigidity of Annie's past. In truth, Annie would begin risking me, wondering if I would stay long enough for her to lean on me. In this lean, Annie's fragments might begin to organize, a bit at a time, allowing neurons between the limbic system of survival (the wolf) to suffer more organization (taming) by the frontal brain. This interior reliability is really the catalyst for story-safety, and for a memory that can first power up with "my story" and then navigate a systems-narrative of "our storying." Because another continually shows up and stands by without intruding, the storying organizes. This is important. We are crucial. But we are not the child's own amalgam of experiences, feeling states, hurts, and nonverbal memories.

For a child, there is no logical separation between the therapist who offers safe relationship and the toys who are vehicles to interacting in this relationship. The toys actually become feeling states that carry the relationship down into the narrow tunnels of implicit memory. There is little to no verbal explanation behind greater implicit acceptance of self and the resulting relief in the child's trust of we together. When the child senses that she has been found, she says, "Come on then. Let's go to where I haven't been understood. Let's see if I can *get* understood." When we talk about implicit memory, we are also talking about implicit reality within the child. Refer to the meaning of implicit: "contained in the nature of something though not readily apparent." Safety and trust in a child's use of relationship is implicit and fluid. Lack of trust is rigid, in need of control (and in need of survival), and disorganized.

In typical healthy development, a child's world of healthy home and family, of perception and meaning making, are going on. Out in the backyard, a small five-year-old builds a nest for the birds so that he might see them better, and speak with them at closer range. It is his understanding of the adage "build it and they will come." A 7 year old works and works in her dollhouse to create the finer details of a room that has everything in it you could possibly wish for. She insists internally that this wish might be useful some day, even as development is pushing her out of these young wish-means-event and toward a more cause-and-event comprehension.

In this deeper level of trust and attachment, the brain responds to and coordinates with another, but is less able to use language. This is the place of art, spiritual icons, images and dreams, where the child enters spontaneously and naturally. The child is fully engaged in the feelings that utter and mutter through the toys. In her writing, *War of the Ancient Dragon*, Laurel Howe tells us that children engage in a natural process which she compares to that of the alchemist. She goes on to explain what we mean by "natural process"- that space in which the child isn't skeptical of the small miracles in a day and doesn't stop to analyze whether or not we are projecting something onto an object (Howe, 2016). The child anticipates something surprising and exciting will happen, without measuring the outcome.

Therapeutic Meaning Making

It is the therapist and the tray, or the room itself, that maintain the containment of the volatile expressions of the child. And if the relationship has been appropriately built, the container holds.

At one point, I let Annie know that the following week we would look at some of the work she had done so far. I had not done this before, nor have I done it since. But the next week she comes in and looks at me guardedly. I offer that this is the day we are going to look at some of the stories she has built. I have chosen only a few sandtray images that were very important, especially those where the wolf is her helper. She is elated! She stands on a chair and dances, again yelling at God, "Do you see that, God—do you see I get to be remembered?! Can you see me here, God, just dancin'!" She can't stop wiggling until I turn on the projector. She watches in attention as we witness her important "history" together.

Annie is amazed that I have collected what she refers to as "story-pictures"; the images she has created in the sandtray. She states, "I have so many stories. So many things have happened. I just had to do all this work, and that's why you're here. What I'm doing is just takin' my time here." Her jubilance nearly overwhelms me. I feel the giddiness of her efforts to believe that

I'm as present as she needs me to be. I want to tell her to get down, be careful. As I move closer to her, I make efforts to find joy with Annie in order to settle us both down together.

Annie's dancing also holds the terrible struggle of staying alert to her experiences. Her behaviors, though intruders to any family that fostered her, are actually keeping the loss of her little brother alive to her. There may have been some unconscious logic as to why Annie had not yet been adopted: perhaps her psychic position is as the story-keeper. The burden of that position had made her quite rigid in who and what rules she would accept as helpful to her.

It often felt as though I worked with a three-year-old armored for battle at any given moment. This readiness showed in her behaviors: ready to whop someone, or pester them. She had her weapons on hand all the time. Somehow, between God, Annie, and myself, we were constructing a beginner's trust that shouted to anyone who would hear that she and her baby brother were finally believed, and in the expectation of that, Annie was beginning to have feelings that shouted as loud as a new baby's cries.

In this space, we move from implicit memory, the interior meaning-maker, to building a safety space so that linkages between two people will occur. Receptivity in the therapeutic relationship, which has no words, holds what was unbearable while it becomes nameable. As these experiences can be thought about, they become *my* experience, and they are *me*. This is the foundation of being found.

And so, the image of Annie's wolf carried the image of Annie's wilderness history until she and I would face the wolf together. Once the wolf became alive, that image carried the duality of Annie's own need for a guard dog and her need to keep memory at bay, of extreme vulnerability from the inside out, and of danger if someone was to reopen her inborn longing to be understood. When she called out to a very large resource, God, to name that she was being re-membered after dis-membering, she brought the real danger into the relationship: that having no one to remember her, she had only scraps of stories.

Annie's process with me stopped when she was adopted out of state. She refused to say goodbye or to make rituals that might help her make this fragile transition. Her need was so great to run toward a family who might take care of her. The new family also resisted participating in transitional requirements. It's very important that any child who has suffered these layers of neglect be given time to transfer loyalties. It's up to the adults to slow transitions down to a crawl, following the child's own cues as to the meanings the child gives such deep change. Annie's move was difficult for me, as I had grown so attached to this spirited little survivor. I couldn't imagine how difficult it might be for her. Her rush to leave brought her wolf further into my landscape. I felt my own attachment prowling around her edges, wanting to have done something more, something less tenuous. I was able to transition Annie into the container of another sandplay therapist in her new hometown.

Memory Fragments

Children have told me fragments of their lives that have no paragraphs to live in. A four-year-old I witnessed could enter a state of panic and meltdown when certain structured routines, such as circle time or lining up, were called. She couldn't manage the morning's circle time, where the children were close to one another, and where her attention needed to remain focused on the teacher's combination of singing and finger play. She simply couldn't rest in the proximity of eight or nine other young children. At one point, with her in my lap, I whispered to her that she might think something bad would happen if I left her in the noisy chaos. *She looked at me without any emotion and said, "There will be a fire and you can't see me."* I held that. At the next parent conference I asked her aunt about any fires in the child's past. "Oh yeah. There was a house fire when she was maybe six months old. It took a bit to reach her crib but she was fine. That was a long time ago." This unintegrated fragment held center for my little friend. It was as if something had stayed cold and unheard, and when her surroundings became noisy, her memory ignited the chaos of whatever had been there to help her. But the image had gone nowhere. It remained in cold storage, disconnected and only appearing suddenly when enough "noise" pushed it to the surface. A long time ago remains now when a felt terror is not given its due.

Remembering

Often enough children have questioned whether I can remember them. What *is* remembering, anyway? Remember and memory share a common root word in the making of language. Remember is "to call to mind; think of again," "to keep [someone] in mind as worthy of consideration or recognition." The dictionary defines memory as "the act of remembering." Memory is the storage container. Remember is the verb, that which brings who we are out of storage and into the dance of two of us, interfacing and resonating and creating something new that was neither of us before. Remembering also calls upon us "to return to an original shape or form after being altered." Remembering is an activity, a return to one's self, if we again want to stretch a bit. When we think about the work of children whose selves have been altered because of wounds and harm done, being remembered through relationship and play is essential. One definition refers to a Norse tale of Mimir, a giant who guards the well of wisdom. If Mimir protects the child's own wisdom, perhaps we play therapists appeal to this giant to release the child's innate path prior to having been altered through wounding. Our own authentic paths reside in our implicit memories and in the meanings we have pinned to our experiences. Playing has the capacity to open the well again. Images in the sand are the bridges into remembering and being found. It's important to play with the images that we find ourselves using over and over, since they are symbolic place-keepers that we might take for granted if we ourselves forget what we're doing with language.

Memory is something we may take for granted. But it is not assumed in a child who has experienced neglect and impoverished attachments. Memory for a child means that someone outside the self is lovingly recording that particular child's self as it grows into a separate individual. It also infers what Winnicott points to when he speaks of playing alone in the presence of another. Here, that points to a child's trust in the reliability of someone outside the self who is simply holding the relationship for two while one of "us" goes rogue for a bit (Winnicott, 1971).

The constructions of memory in children entails some mixture of actual event(s), listening to others or looking at photos that describe the event(s), and subjective imagination. The most important factor in the equation of memory in children is its charged feeling. Recall that explicit memory is not yet playing any major harmonic in the creation of self. So the greater the charged fear (e.g., being lost emotionally, being confused), the more the memory isolates from view (Fernyhough, 2012). At some point a charged experience is no longer available to memory except by its attribute of smell, noises, the color of someone's hair, the lifting-off sense of being above one's body.

Annie's wolf may well be thought of as something merely imagined. If so, we haven't gone far enough in our understanding. This discounts the significance of the task of this image. The wolf may play the constant in a young child's otherwise unwilling memories which include both events and feeling states being overwhelmed. To cut through these protectors with premature language or solution-focused interventions is likely to feel like yet another invasion. Allowing the images to emerge as the child experiences the connecting links of another person will gradually update the child's sense of trust and reliance. The image is the information bearer, we might say, that activity that dips into the storage container of memory, puts flesh and bone on a feeling, and pushes that feeling-as-image into the space between therapist and child.

We therapists are the gatekeepers of this gradual trust building: how much, when and where to press on, and when simply to stand by. In children such as Annie, we are beginning again, taking the feeling states as they are and slowly creating ways to tolerate them while Annie builds the trust required for her to create a constant self-image. Over time Annie will learn to calm those states that the wolf protects her from. In addition, her behaviors are telling us just how a wolf behaves when that primitive self is in charge of protection. The wolf image is a stand-in to any sense of internal order that Annie had achieved. It cannot do the job of knowing Annie, of wiring her up to an outside modulator when her feelings overwhelm her. The wolf can only be a singular resource that stands ready, an armor of fierce wildness that fosters her less relational efforts to remember herself.

Annie had not yet learned to trust, which is a pre-one-year-old process. While other developmental milestones of creating a sense of self continued on, Annie required an other who would reside as a surrogate in the place of an attending parent. Trust itself is the dynamic that allows an unveiling of old wounds and then reaches into very young development to revise and transform the mysteries of "us" and the implied meanings we have given to that us.

When we think about the importance of memory in young children, it works best to not-think. Thinking only carries us to the point of discussing what memory is. But reasoning won't capture the effort of the child in need of being remembered. Staying out of logic keeps a wide-angle lens in our own tracking. A more fluid state addresses the braiding effects of imagination and story composition. At some point in the process of co-construction, the child will move toward a sort of evaluation of events with their feeling states. That is the time to bring in historic photos and create timelines of that child's pathway. To do this too soon sends the message to the child that he or she is too difficult to carry into a mutual remembering place. When we are timely in our introduction to remembering, the child will be able to accept the stories that belong to her with less fear that the failures were her fault. Following deep work in safe play, the container that has been built from image-making in sandtray or in art therapy will hold the feelings so that they don't fall back into the child's unwitnessed developing sense of self.

What has gone missing, and therefore what has abandoned the child to an isolated and unregulated space, is this raw truth—that no one has carried that child in his or her mind. No one has held this child safely, organizing relationship into a complex pathway that builds upon itself, onto a map or matrix that supports the child's self as it moves and safely wanders about within another's reflective presence. Having had no one to wire-up with, the child has too few experiences of being special to anyone. Symbols like the wolf are wordless secret meanings. Faith in these symbols guide us in the work. Having faith in the child and the child's own pathways will find the child's self. Understanding brings about remembering, and remembering, to the child, is being found.

CHAPTER 3
Jamal: Development and Trust

I worked a long time with a grandmother who had adopted her grandson, Jamal, at 10 months of age, after the baby's parents were both unable to be available to the baby. Around age 4 he drastically increased biting and scratching her. It seemed she had reached her own tolerance of these aggressions. Between her limits and Jamal's increasing exposure to other environments (and therefore, much higher anxiety) the two were in an emotional power struggle of survival proportions. As I listened to the grandmother's history report, I heard that she believed that her early intercession had saved this child from ongoing pain. She had surely been his most profound intervention. Yet, without meaning to, she had forfeited his own intrinsic meanings of those first 10 months. As Jamal became more alert to the demands of trust and depending on other adults, this little guy kept returning to his baby times. There was too little resource, too little wiring-up, when he found himself attempting to trust new adults. And Grandma's connections weren't there in his early experiences, either. So he gave his increasing anxieties over to her. It was as if he was aggressively shouting, "Find me! I'm so scared!" Meanwhile, she was retreating. No language was helpful here.

Let us jump into the meaning of the word development for a minute. In music, development "elaborates a theme of harmonic variations to render into visibility." In photography: "to process, in order to render an image more visible." To develop is "to strengthen," "to become affected with," "to transform" (American Heritage Dictionary, 1992). It is crucial to hang on to these markers rather than what can become a linear arrow that pierces time and space as a human being develops. We are not linear, and our development is not linear. We are all in our own individuation processes that render our images more visible and more usable to us. We struggle to be in harmonious relationship and to be affected by the intimate efforts of others. Here we are more able to find the child who enters our lives, needing us to guide her toward images becoming realities that nourish her, and us.

What occurred in the development of the infant reflects in play and in play therapy. This greatly helps us understand who we are seeing in the playroom. While the child in our room might be 4 or 5, we re-enter the youngest realms of attachment, dependency, and attunement. Context is necessary for understanding this process. We need to have some bracing to lean on when we scamper too far into the interior of the child's self.

Creation of the Child

What creates a child? Winnicott states, "At the theoretical start, the baby lives in a dream world while awake" (Winnicott, 1971). A child is born into a body, and then it interacts in its world to create its realness. The mother essentially dreams the baby into a separate self. A good enough mother will endure her world being intruded upon by the pull to envision her baby forward. Psychology sometimes calls this symbiosis, in which attachment is embedded.

In the beginning of life, the newborn is all subject. The real and the imaginative are one and the same thing. Being subject, the infant is the creator of all. Connection is being made and then repeatedly updated and renewed through the baby's recognition of the caregiver's smell, voice, touch. These repetitive sensations come to be the map of what safety feels like. The baby's body is like a highly tuned antenna. The baby's senses include the skin as a powerful relational informant. All this is profoundly infused with the parent's feeling states which, when congruent, offer the attunement the baby requires. This will surface as a form of nonverbal communication far into the future as being remembered, being found. Here, in this beginning, the intersections of attunement, language and memory are bumping about finding their interlaced placement within an inner map. This map builds a future potentially organized and separate human being.

What a child experiences in the environment is understood through the pathways of the central nervous system. The central nervous system is the primary player, which responds to information that is perceived through the senses (Peterson, 2014). In domestic violence, for example, the child's senses receive the intensity and volume in sound coupled with the feeling of physical threat and (lastly) the emotional impact of threat and fear. The area of the brain that perceives in this manner is the limbic system. Located in the more primitive brain parts, particularly in the brain stem, this system governs the second-by-second filter response of the senses. This is an essential dynamic for survival in anyone, especially those who are most vulnerable. Often repeated threats instill their own neuropathways, and, if not regulated and moved into narration, the child's experiences will remain un-thought and dysregulating – in present time—as triggers.

I ask Grandma to go back with Jamal, literally to provide connecting exchanges that might introduce her deep care into his "baby-map." I encourage her to rock him and to offer a bottle or some comforting drink that might connect the two of them in its shared action. Jamal has no problem with the new morning and evening ritual of rocking together while drinking Kefir from a bottle. At first, Grandma reports that she felt embarrassed to do this. But she soon relaxes into Jamal's own enjoyment of being with her in this closeness. Eye-to-eye contact during these periods offers acceptance, rapport, and the wiring-up that Jamal needs. As his physical aggressions decreases, little by little, we add other connecting options that all focus on Grandma's efforts to be present to Jamal's infant hurts. Jamal himself wants to wear diapers for a bit, and with great trepidation, Grandma okays certain times as "diaper times." He really has a sense of his own limits here, going back to having an infant's needs while simultaneously wearing his own underwear. Over time, Grandma's willingness to establish her loving care in the landscape of Jamal's early infancy resettles his aroused systems. She is able to guide him from the lost developmental windows where trust had been wanting, toward being his 4-year-old self.

The infant's emotions are entirely externally regulated by the primary caregiver. This makes sense, as the infant's focus is grounded by the limbic system. This isn't to say that no affect exists or that the baby is a set of neuro-firings. Not at all. It does, however, underscore our awareness that the baby's caregiver holds the full impact of the infant's feeling states. The infant is at the mercy of the caregiver to mold and develop its internal system of regulation. At first, all the baby can offer is a cry to let the caregiver know that an empathic wiring-up is necessary. The caregiver is the responsible and trust-worthy person who needs to estimate the baby's needs. Slowly but surely the wiring-up takes on an internal and subjective meaning to the baby. It is interesting to note that the roots of the words *self* and *secure* are the same. The Latin word *securus*, from the same root, means "away from" and thus *securus* means "away from worry."

To be clear, the baby's, and the young child's, regulation is located within the relationship of reciprocity and trust. Where the give and take of feelings, understandings, missed cues are all met with an adult's openness, the baby learns regulation over a period of years. This cannot be overstated. This is the relational dynamic that initiates and maintains what we might discuss too lightly: self-regulation, self-awareness that modulates behaviors—all those underpinnings that define a healthy adult. And crucially, this relational dynamic must be secured enough for future learning to take place. The rudder that steers all understanding of the baby's personhood is this: the baby *is* the relationship. She will come from this mutuality, into a self. Every child in this narration will show us their own pathways toward this effort.

In the very young infant, rage is evident and normal. It functions as a kind of survival drive, alerting the primary parent to sudden high levels of unrestrained need. The parent is accountable to constant and consistent response, bringing required satisfaction, which includes her devotion. For the first several months of life, the baby cannot self-regulate states of "narcissistic rage." The infant's distresses will drive him into extremely high levels of arousal which are beyond his own capacity to sustain (Delahooke, 2019; Schore, 1994). The adult is the sole modulator and is attuned to her child's needs.

This symbiosis gradually shifts, while the mother remains awake to the infant's separate needs. The mother holds the brooding beginnings of the infant while navigating the potential separateness of two individuals, the mother and the baby. This indefinable sense of oneness within twoness is the new mother's task, and this establishes the trust from within the baby's self that will usher in a healthy separateness in the first year of life.

Trust as a Developmental Task

Trust is a core truth that lies in the body of the infant. Those sounds, smells, touches, and being held organize the baby's own neural body. Embodiment is defined as "giving form to;

to represent in material form"; and "to make part of a system or whole; incorporate" (American Heritage Dictionary, 1992). Embodiment and trust are partners in a sort of spiritual melding that materializes in a separate being who is at the same time part of a larger system and a larger story. The infant carries in her creation, her development, the makings of a body, a separating self. She is the form, the representation in a body with its own neurons and history, that must organize a story of self over time. And all this is dependent on (bound to) the system in which this separating self lives and grows. Organization utterly depends on the parent's own capacity to remain organized in feeling tones, responses, and internal stressors. These tonal organizing narrations are the beginning stories the baby attends to and records in implicit memory. We can rightly say that these are the sounds and feelings that are the baby until the baby forms some amount of embodiment that facilitates a separation of self from the mother.

Care is not merely physical. The infant, in states of all-calm or all-rest, absorbs care through all senses and feelings. There are minimal stoppages to outbreaks of "all of me is upset!" When the baby cries from a disruption of that calm, that little being is brought back by the mother, to a place of calm. The parent registers the baby's hiccup in a field of unity and responds to the baby sufficiently enough to bring the baby back into that unity.

This kind of trust is perhaps particular to the caregiver-infant state. We are able to compare it to many other states of being, but in itself it is something that, if held deeply and thoroughly enough, we are meant to leave. This second emergence, which Winnicott names hatching, pushes each of us toward separateness and the initiation of an existential self (Winnicott, 1971). We are in this unified state in order to trust the environment enough to welcome our separateness. What a beautiful dance this is. It has two partners, although the baby only registers one for a small period of time. And then she hatches out because she has the foundation around her to begin that inner growth we call the self. The first core reliability—the trustworthiness—is in this deeply attuned state out of which the baby herself initiates being and safety. The parent offers the baby recognition that being omnipotent for a few months is fine! We caregivers are willing to hold the world while assuming the giant task of keeping that world safe until this particular entity internalizes the safety we represent. To the baby, the world is her body, and the skin to that world is the loving parent. Trust and safety enter the baby through the limbic system, which is constructing a home, a place to live, for this infant.

Gifts of the Limbic System

So often, we discuss the limbic system in human beings in the context of trauma. This system deserves recognition as the key player in the baby's first developmental processes. The limbic system is engaged in feeding, aggression, body needs, and the complex resonance between mother and baby. When we track the baby's signals and signs to his vital parent connection, we already perceive the baby's story forming. We are able to gain insight into the baby's very own communication and his temperament through how he responds and reacts to his primary safety connections and his reliance in the environment. The baby's cues are rich with that unique baby's initiating mythos. Relationship holds trust, without which we cannot be whole. The infant is utterly reliant on his mother's intuitive containment. What we have here in the service to trust, is the adult's full use of her own limbic system, her own gut instincts.

What is much more difficult to articulate is the vitality of this mutual state. The parent uses what trackers call wide-angle vision, the same intuitive focus that honors the less visible and brings what is scanned into awareness as a possibility. The baby's cues are possibilities, signals that the parent assesses in her deeper gut-knowing. Because the infant is unconditionally wiring to the primary parent, there are no checks and balances in place. When the mother dysregulates, the baby's brain synchronistically registers overload, and the baby must protect itself by dropping away from the wiring. Too much of this kind of withdrawal and dropping away becomes a trauma pattern.

The limbic system is central in the mother's constant invitation to the baby's cues. As the mother attends to her baby's cues, she is simultaneously claiming this little one as the one who receives her devotion. Mother and baby are in one story, building meaning until the baby has the holistic stamina to begin the long journey of becoming a subjective story of her own. The nuances here are those of the newborn mammal who must learn to survive in a "wilderness" of sorts, that of society itself. Before any of that, ideally before any challenges to the core, the baby inhales the mother's own resources as belonging to both, as one unit.

In yet another paradox, the key dynamic of regulation has its tensions. The good enough parent (Winnicott, 1971) is one who can receive the infant's un-regulating. As that un-wired ache in the infant reaches into the adult, in the mutual "us" space, the mother intuits where this discomfort lives. Here is the use of the gut as informer. If the baby is tired, and his fussing scales upward to crying, it is this adult who comprehends that the world has gotten too heavy, and it is time to seek the simplicity of one set of eyes. And then she repairs the gap that had expressed itself through sensate and feeling states. This space she devotedly enters is not about who is regulating, but precisely about the dance of co-regulating. It takes two to have a relationship that, breathingly, is alive and adjusts its emotional heart rate for two.

Winnicott states that around 8-9 months, the infant is "hatched," a sort of second birth in which the infant begins the process of becoming an individual (Winnicott, 1971). There is a growing recognition in the baby of what is "not me," thereby making space for what "is me." At this juncture the self begins. This is a long and complex journey. Understanding these developmental markers is vital when we are with a hurting child and wondering who is in our presence. If those markers were not achieved, we will return to those gaps in play therapy. It is imperative that we are able to accept this task, through both training and through the capacity to understand the unified "us" state. The gaps are quite specific in their effort to discover the child in an arena that had originally left them feeling too unsafe or unwired-up to accomplish the tasks of that stage.

Therapeutic rapport returns to this landscape of possibilities over and over. Working with young children who are wounded, we ourselves must discover that wide-angle lens within. We need to have done enough inner work that we can rely on the wisdom of the gut, the intuitive understanding that takes the child's hand and goes back to these earlier spaces. If we are with a 6-year-old, for instance, who is now in foster care, enough trust in the current therapy relationship will urge the child to go back and find out what it feels like to depend on an adult's presence. Needs that had been shuttered down for lack of resonance, now open up again. The limbic system is the most active dynamic as the child tries again to be seen, opens up again to possibilities rather than rigid protectors.

Jamal enters kindergarten. He now has a bit of calming in his system. Nonetheless, the school environment proves to be too intense for him. He returns to his aggressive behaviors at home, while somatic problems now appear. Jamal's stomach hurts nearly every morning. We add his teacher to our team. She is compassionate toward Jamal's challenges. Grandma and the teacher create a looser schedule for Jamal's appearance in the morning, lifting some of the burden off of Jamal's own sensitive neuro-system. The teacher adds in some allowances, like Jamal going to a quiet place in the room when he feels upset. These added soothers seem to help Jamal bring his trust of Grandma forward, toward his teacher. Jamal's impulsivity is not only about his turbulent beginnings. Temperament is also engaged. Jamal's sensitivities become more understood during his kindergarten year, paving the way for a little more flexibility in school. Academics comes easily for him. It will be the emotional development that needs steady attention.

We often approach the limbic system as a part of the brain that must be tamed, decreased in its strength of non-verbal, first-hand signs. In truth, this system is what allows us to see through another's eyes and ears. It reveals, as if to an inner eye, when to stop, when to ponder, when to run. It is the signatory to that which is safe enough to remain in a mutual field, an inter-play of two with no one being in power. And so important to the work and play of child therapy, it is the tap-dancer in the field of imagination. When we move toward overly taming the child's instincts, we are quieting the great element of imagining, the creation of something out of "nothing" and the trust that the nothing will respond.

This system of alert/response/react isn't meant to run the day. Yet, psychology has swung too far in its efforts to train rather than to trust. Trusting the other allows that other a place to stand while the child offers the real information we will need in our own responses. If our responses are gathered from our own executive function, we are in fact thrusting our own government onto the child's needs, letting her know how to proceed from our own rules rather than listening for the child's sense of truth. Truth is in there: Remember, the child is bound by a story of her own, and her authorship will assist us soon enough in working together for shared understanding. It is dependent on the adult to regulate communications in order that the child might articulate what is occurring internally. The adult trusts that at the core of every individual's survival is a need to be understood. The limbic system pushes and tugs at how to find this mutual space.

Trust Reprised

The word trust is such a large space. It can mean "to become firm, solid, steadfast," which applies to a baby's evolution toward a self (American Heritage Dictionary, 1992). Trust, in its definition, includes faith, authenticity. Trust also partners with safety. It is worth wondering and wandering, connecting these filaments one to another, because within this web, we begin to recognize and treasure what it takes to gain wholeness for ourselves. And what it takes is thoroughly located in relationship, in an "us" state until interior shifts call upon "us" to recognize "me-and-you."

Healthy development means that the loving adult is able to enter "imaginatively and yet accurately into the thoughts and feelings and hopes and fears of her baby; also to allow the baby to do the same to the mother" (Winnicott, 1971). The word "allow" implies a certain level of awareness: If we are to allow something, it can indicate that there are options, and we choose to allow the baby to enter our interior feelings and hopes and fears. A tacit underpinning here is that adults have some understanding of what a relationship truly needs so that they will choose to allow this interchange. This is clearly just what our task is as therapists: to enter "imaginatively and yet accurately into the thoughts and feelings and hopes and fears of our child," (Winnicott, 1971) also to allow the child to do the same to ourselves. It refers to dynamics: of being found trustworthy, available to the child's disruptures and longings without any compromise or discount on our end of that dynamic.

As a child's brain struggles and triumphs over an overwhelming ebb and flow of feelings minus her thinking, other deeper layers of development are also hard at work. There is, after all, a private self that is approaching us, even as we hear the high-spirited efforts and creativity of "No!" in the toddler and "I didn't do that" in the pre-schooler. These exercises in power and self-determination bring on board the incredible force of language and its ability to both dominate another and to create connection through being understood. Learning to voice who we are and what we feel builds, over time, a bridge from the right-sided brain of feeling states to our own "executive function," the CEO that maintains order even in feelings that are overwhelming. The beginnings of this internal bridge occur within and alongside the very young human being's attunement to another who for some period of time, is that bridge for this budding evolution. Language becomes the carrier of affect at the same time the child is learning to regulate. While all this amazing activity is occurring, the earliest attunement and cuing from the parent is the fertile ground of language and wiring up to words-as-symbols of our own inner life force.

As Jamal experiences his grandmother's full presence and feels his nonverbal needs being loveable, he begins to relax. This is not a quiet process. Grandma continues to call in for coaching when she feels herself push away from Jamal. She wants his aggression and impulsivity to go away. Those behaviors trigger worries in herself about "angry men." We work away at finding out possibilities of what Jamal needs to say through his behaviors. Grandma's own story, of disappointment in her son as a father, of dread for baby Jamal, and of the risk she has taken to be a parent now, are all her story. She needs to hear herself as Jamal calls her to find him.

How do we who offer support to the young child's interior mapwork begin to understand how the child has put together experience, fact, and memory? Our first commitment is to this underlayer of each child's self, where verbal language is not yet the strongpoint of communication. Coming from the place of feelings and how those feelings are all subject for the child, the match and congruence of communication will be in the use of images and symbols, on one hand, and body states on the other. And congruence for us as therapists is often how our bodies feel, rather suddenly, during our time with a child. Are we rather suddenly sleepy? What wants to phase out? Are we itching to get up, walk around? What needs movement? We can at least console ourselves that we have successfully wired-up to the child's embodied self! It certainly is not that the child does not yet communicate well: It is because the communication used is not thoroughly hampered by logic. When we speak about children being at home in play, we are simultaneously speaking about their communication with their environment. We walk alongside the child's own close company with their inner sensations.

When working and playing with a child who has been separated from her parent and has suffered chronic neglect, one important task is to build the mapwork, perhaps for the first stabilizing time. Begin with those wiring-up cues: smell, touch, taste. When the adopting mother puts almond-scented lotion on both her child and herself, commenting on they will smell the same all day, and she repeats this over and over, the wiring in the child begins again, hunting through the senses for the attuning other. And remember, "self" and "secure" come from the same root: below the surface of what we see.

The Role of Language

One key strand that is strengthening this underground web is language. Over time, language will serve a vital purpose. Over a period of years, words organize our feeling states, and that interior order will then stabilize the space between us. It will never replace the meanings we give to that space. Recall that us-space of the infant. We are meant to individuate and become our own boss, our own author. The profound truth here is that while we work away at the growing internal stabilization of self, the requirement of attachment never decreases. We move out of dependent, to inter-dependent. And this inter-space requires communication the more safely separate we become. Language is the internet of communication and of wiring together, the fast-processing symbols that travel back and forth between us in the fine filaments we share. Language derives from symbol-representatives that we co-author and that are rewarded with the nuances in someone's mirroring eyes. These symbols will build from trust, from the child's perceptions of having been seen and understood throughout earlier strong modes of communication.

Language serves as the mediator, the dynamic that encodes one's own meaning-making, files it into a subjective (me-driven) order, and builds a history from this authorship. The history of ourselves prior to this mediator is enveloped in sensations and feeling states. Though they do not register in word order, these states are held as a vital story-of-origin, where the impetus for a separate self is stored in a much larger platform of knowing an *us* in order to find a *me.* The momentum to become me, a self that enjoys its empowerment, originates in the trust and reliability I have had in you as my parent, and in us as having danced safely together. We might say that each of us has our very own creation myth that, for better and worse, serves as the boldness of our own evolution. Language is alive and stunning when we keep it in its subjective development, as the result of image-building rather than the best or go-to resource for communication. When we believe words will create understanding with little relational meaning in place, we are in error. This helps us in our works with parents, who might not have patience enough to understand or tolerate when their child seems to suddenly talk "baby talk," or goes silent, as Delilah did. The child returns to the impetus for language, and the safer use of somatic sensations ("Mommy, my tummy hurts" when another day of school is imminent), or intense eruption of feelings, when the going gets too tough. The origin of that yearning to be a strong separate self is the home base within. We circle back and touch the core of what we mean when we say the word attachment.

In the rapprochement crisis that Mahler (1975) speaks of, this struggle moves into the relationship *between* the two, rather than a unified feeling state. The child initiates a very long practice period of taking in the capacity to self-soothe through experiences of hyper-arousal. Self soothing is learned by being soothed. Hyper-arousal and the baby's own beginning self can be seen when the baby looks away from the highly charged face of the mother, pauses, and then returns to find connection. The baby in a healthy relationship also utilizes strong facial responses that alert the mother to her attunement, when is it enough, too much, not enough. As the baby begins to take in a separateness that is still safe, she also begins the struggle and success of increasing autonomy. All of this takes place under the secured umbrella of the parent. The parent will support and modulate stronger feelings like anger and aggression, which are in the service of separation and trust. Mahler addresses the rapprochement phase of the 2 to 3-year-old as "travelling from a belief in his own and in his parents' omnipotence [to] autonomous functioning." She states also "throughout the whole course of separation-individuation one of the most important developmental tasks of the evolving ego is that of coping with the aggressive drive in the face of the gradually increasing awareness of separation" (Mahler, 1975). The young child creates a sense of deep safety and security, of being taken care of, out of a gradual connection/autonomy regulation. From this deep place of trust, self-esteem grows. What a precarious process these first years of life involve.

As this dynamic of word usage increases, we cannot make the mistake of believing that the young child who states, "I *hate* you!" knows the meaning of that aggression. Here the child tries on power to see what happens to her own intense feelings, not to see if we like being hated. When we remain connected and clear about the task, success has been that the child tried out power as an undiluted feeling. And nobody disappeared. Nobody took the power away. Instead, the child's practice of aggression gets understood. What is so important is that parents, teachers, and therapists help the child learn about our less-than-liked human aspects like anger, fear, and hating, and the use of dominating words. If we use domination to mollify the child's practice moments, the child learns that he is powerless. This power over others is what we have taught. As an adult, the child selects from an either/or pattern: either powerlessness or dominance.

The safer the child feels in his primary relationship(s), the more self-recognition he can apply to the next tasks. The fulcrum of development in the very young child is a profound long-lasting transitional period which follows on the heels of emotional regulation rehearsals. The child, for the first time, must begin to endure holding the tension of opposites, in particular the polar opposite of pulling away from significant others in order to build and integrate a self. The fulcrum of development in the preschooler is a profound transitional period. The child is moving out of the primal relationship of mother, toward a social context. Any individual who works thoroughly on wholeness must be able to say "no" and mean it when he is learning about personal power and personal protection.

The child must aggress outward for the first time as an individualized self, holding the tension of being dependently attached in order to move away. The nonlinear paradox here is that in order to move outward, one must be held. Ultimately, one must expand and separate so that one may notice and identify one's own self. The child as "center of the world" must gradually integrate the world into her center: become civilized. In this give and take of individuation lies confidence, self esteem, and the ability to be curious about one's self and the other rather than either/or. This process of individuation is here in its plainest form, and perhaps, therefore, is most profoundly vulnerable, in this "first attempt."

The Child's Form of Knowing

I have been watching 5-year-old Johnny make circuit board drawings, images of what his father does for a living. I say, "I'm impressed by how much you've learned." Johnny looks into me for a while, then goes back to his work. "I really just know everything already. I just don't have time to tell you it all. I haven't really learned that much." Johnny has quietly invited me to change my tune, to discover something together that he "just knows" somewhere inside.

As we receive and are receptive to each child's implicit meanings, the child grows more able to trust this relational environment, and to consider the messages of two people who are interactive. This is a most important paradox: As we adults hunt for and find the child's own meanings that motivate his words and behaviors, we are in those exchanges that build the child's trust in himself, his own reservoirs of confidence and self-esteem. We are not catering to the child. We are instead finding the congruent needs and messages while we hear and respond to the child. Discovering what the child means and perceives does not mean that we are to obey. We are meant to understand, and to assist the child in finding out how to be successful in communicating his needs and wants.

To "know" is defined as "to perceive or understand as truth, to have something fixed in memory—to understand from experience, to be aware of meaning" (American Heritage Dictionary, 1992). Is Johnny saying he has his own awareness of meaning, thank you very much, and my own ignorant statement of "you've learned so much" intrudes on that knowingness? In the child's experience of play lies the creation of meaning. Knowledge happens as we ourselves connect what we already know with what is going to be experienced or learned (Flynn, 1991).

The play of the child is not what the adult perceives as learning, per se. There is little to no separation between learning, revealing, and play for the child. The adult too often approaches the child's world-making with a sense of knowing what the child needs to learn, and therefore lays upon the child's metaphoric meanings a logical and linear comprehension. In these times, we intrude in the child's metaphoric and meaning-making expressions with our need to be the authority who makes sense. Often enough I have fallen prey to pressures from the child's own environments or to my own tiredness. I step away from tracking the child and into a hope that what I have to offer will make sense to both of us. This type of situation presents when a teacher sends an urgent email that says, "this morning was very difficult." I might ask the child what happened at school this morning rather than waiting out the child's own need to reach emotional safety, bring her heart rate down, and then inform me about what has thrown her off. I may have a little less to share with the teacher on that day, but I will have succeeded in a consistent effort to calm the child's own meaning-maker enough that she will make sense to herself. The child is already somewhere in her story and in the continued creation of her story. A wounded child cannot find herself in her story. The symbols she uses will locate her. She has her own internal rhythm that helps her feel safe with me, and no amount of quickening the process will reveal the truths she hunts for. It is important to choose whether or not it helps to introduce the morning's events. Sense-making and meaning-making might be addressed as two different routes of discovery. What would change if adults approached the child with curiosity that wonders, in the child's play, what she is creating and expanding in her inner world of knowing.

The child's own core, her sense of self, is bonded internally to early parenting. Strong interactions reinforce who the parent recognizes the child to be and who the parent disallows the child to be. Parents show the child who he is through their behaviors over what they accept and what they will not tolerate in the child.

Jamal: Development and Trust

The parents' acceptance and refusal toward the child crops and trims the child, showing who this child can and cannot be. That is, by relating to the child as though he is such and such and ignoring other aspects of him as if they do not exist, the parents disconfirm (Laing, 1962) the relational existence of those aspects of the child's self that they ignore. This gradual disconnection of the child's unwanted behaviors from the core self of the child is relationally nonnegotiable. Continued trimming away of what doesn't fit in the parent's eye, is intrinsic to the existence of developmental (relational) trauma. Such trauma is typically cumulative. What was not acceptable to the primary parent(s) is no longer acceptable to the child's core self, either. The developing child must find and then update ways to keep out any aspects of self that were originally unacceptable (Bromberg, 2011).

The question we logically thinking adults have responsibility for is this: How might we enter the child's perceptions and feeling-states from the pathway of the child's self, one who is creating meaning, rather than one who must be trained? This entry is vital; otherwise we invade the child's world with our own conditions and definitions. An adult who longs to help the child make sense prematurely has intruded and betrayed the child's creation myth, which continues to be written in the meaning-making self of the child. Adopted children are very susceptible to this dynamic. Many adopting parents need help to build the narration that will assist their new family to remain close to the child's own story. Going too quickly into how this new family is the child's forever family may easily forfeit the child's ability to *find out* about this family. Internally, he may feel he must throw away his story because now there is a new story, a better one according to the affect being related to him.

I worked with a little guy whose behaviors were completely feral. In his first 4 years he had lived with his mentally ill mom. Now he would be adopted. We worked hard on building his trust. The new mom was attentive to both using new experiences that she and I discussed, and being consistent in her responses and behaviors. About 10 months into the work, this little guy just collapsed in the play and began sobbing. I held him while he made contact with his grief. He was able to tell me, "I can't remember my mama! Where is my mama? What is her face?!" It didn't matter which mama he meant, although I knew from his sorrow that he was losing the loyalty to his birth mom. I called his adoptive mom, and he talked with her on the phone. They agreed she would come right over, right now. They cuddled on the couch until he nodded that he would remember this mother's face until after work. This touching scene has helped to inform me about grief and what it must feel like to such a young child. His internal hurdle was held safely by the new mama, while he grieved that he was losing sight of 4 years of another mama.

When we are able to enter through the child's own gate, wiring-up, we enter the child's emotional and meaningful place as witnesses and trustworthy guides who help the child make sense of potentially overwhelming feelings. So does this mean that the child is playing at mock combat, hunting, or evasion? No. The child plays at imagination, creating images not available to the senses; he plays at fantasy, creating and remaking the world to his desire. The figures, with their fantastical functions and the child's imaginal additions, become the heroic ideal by imitating and replicating significant actions and so assuming the champion's power over the world.

Aggression

"Just sharks are going to be in here [in the tray]. The people are going to be little, and the sharks are going to be BIG. The boats are gonna try to run over the sharks. I'm a shark, and my dad is going to try to run over me in a boat... ALL the boats are

Jamal: Development and Trust

Dad. This [anchored] one is him, too. It can't move. The ones that move have alarms that go off when they hit sharks. I'm goin' to have a baby boat. The babies are driving the baby boat. My [big] brother's the babies, and I'm all the sharks. Everybody's afraid of me. The sharks come back to life if they're hurt up. Glug glug. (Buries a boat.) It should'a had a shark alarm."

There is so much aggression here. Underneath, there is a story of helplessness, and the fear of one's overly strong feelings. Maybe this 4-year-old is enraged at his dad's behaviors, and there is no one to help him out. Being a shark is helpful. This child worked these themes over and over, until it was safe enough first to be very helpless, and then to create a central power that had some highly useful options.

Right here is the core of what adults must enter into: What can the child tell us she knows, in order that we might experience our "aha" for having discovered that particular child's knowing. Here is the link-up, the attunement itself, the pearl that words scuttle around and do not quite settle in. It is about exploring together, being curious together while the child offers a meaning that most often is not to be found in the way we adults believe we are communicating. That is the link-up the child requires, and, finding its presence, she agrees to learn from us. The child understands that the adult is holding a space for the child to poke around in, to explore in images and scents and a kaleidoscope of memory fragments that haven't yet been beaded together for a stable "Oh! That's me!" grasp. It is the adult response to the child's intentions, not merely to his actions, which helps the child place his needs and wishes into perspective. That perspective becomes bound together, like paragraphs on a page, as the adult remains devotedly curious, waiting for the child's next inner-to-outer images-into-ideas-and-thoughts. The area of control for the child remains within his range of action while remaining dependent on the caring adult for increased comprehension.

The toddling and preschool years see the child proceeding toward an enduring ego stability. This does not mean stability and the stamina to hold "me" steadily. These years are research and practice years: working on an intermittent, not-yet-enduring sense of self. The child, with her neurology of relationship dynamics, strong feelings, safety needs, real and pretend, is constantly making adjustments and shifts internally. Think about an author deep inside who is cutting and pasting words, phrases, and paragraphs so that they belong more evenly where they are placed. The safer a child feels, the more she can absorb this growing "me" base, and the more likely it becomes that she will reach a place to sort the imagined threats from real dangers. In this process, the child will regain some measure of self-esteem.

Aggression results in behaviors that overwhelm and confuse most adults, whose reactions confront what is good and not-good in the child. Through this lens, the child's aggression must be corrected rather than understood. A major difficulty is the adult creating a good-and-bad basis before the child has reached developmental milestones to remain connected and learn from the parent's position. There's no place to grow this information other than to feel "I'm bad," which impinges on trusting the adult.

As with all crucial milestones within the young child, opposing forces are meant to be contained while the child grows into them and learns about them. Opposing forces work away from within, creating pairs of opposites (Samuels, 1985). This labor for a separate sense of thought and perceiving creates a new product: the conscience (Samuels, 1985). Conscience is that recognition of good and not-good, and the desire to act toward goodness. The child experiments through play, extending his awareness through images of good and bad, and feeling his way into this new place emotionally. Emotions, not the objective reasoning of later years, speak to the child. His imagination, which weaves the telling of his emotions of himself as "explanations," gives him the possibility of effecting change. In this play space, working interiors into images, the child builds what we most hope for: esteem, personal trust, and trust in the world that means my own small self can cause change.

To aggress means to "start an attack or a quarrel; a hostile action or behavior." A root meaning to "aggress" is "ghredh," which means "to walk, go" or "a step, stage, degree" (American Heritage Dictionary, 1992). Playing with images, the young child is now stepping out, going forth. To step out, one may need to quarrel with the past, push against, perhaps create enough tension so as to move away from an old way or construct. The thing is, *we* are the past. We are the old construct that has been the safe-enough base. And yet, in this momentous thrust at growth, we are also what is old, becoming history. If we have done a good-enough job, we are held in the history and in the story of the child's self.

A 3-year-old, when told firmly, "No, it really is time to help pick up toys," states with power, "You just wait! You just wait until I grow up and you grow down!" To aggress is to be hostile. Hostile points to "host"– "one who entertains guests; a guest, a host, a stranger" (American Heritage Dictionary, 1992). Who is the guest the child may be entertaining? – a new self; a newness who is perhaps quite threatening to entertain as a guest? One who will topple all that has been safe, nestled in the parent's attunement? Returning to an earlier developmental requirement to learn about the way opposites function within feeling-states, the definition we are tracking continues. What is the interplay of opposites here: hostility/entertainment, stranger/guest, push against/walk toward. The invitation to stretch, to become wiser and more self-confident, rests in part in a growing comprehension that polar tensions are not resolved through separating what is good from what is bad. At risk of stepping into thin air, the child here in this long transitional space must master that very tension of opposites, as host to the new self, that guest. Attached to the primal relationship of mothering, the child aggresses into the unknown, pushes and expands into a social self that must learn, over time and experiential relationship, to leave home. The beginning of adulthood is hidden right here, in a very long stage of a child's expansion and growth. This is, then, development, a baby's trust being made use of to become, over time, the adult trust in you-and-me that makes full use of this mutuality to one another in healthy and ever-expanding possibilities. "Reciprocal states of responsibility" may be one great working definition of inter-dependence.

The young child will have internalized mothering love for himself, the child, which is Erikson's "basic trust" phase (Erikson, 1994). This trust is hopefully enduring enough, good enough for the child to risk realizing his anxieties and frustrations through play and through expressive behavior. Not perfect, but good enough. The young child wants what he wants immediately, which preserves the newly discovered self-identity of the toddler. But he also, in the dynamics of trust, heartfully depends on approval and love and struggles between this crucial need and those immediate demands from this developmental creation of self and of ego (Delahooke, 2019). This peculiar, nonmental effort occurs through play, where it is safe to incorporate the emotions involved gradually, working out the problem by taking turns between the roles of the bad child, the evil parent, the hero. The adult response toward the child's emotional incorporation of this problem is crucial. Dominating tension appears as aggression throughout this passage of development. The child's great effort to internalize a new self is dependent on the adult's recognition of the seriousness of this work-play. The degree of moral goodness (conscience) the child internalizes is dependent on the adult's safe containment of the child's core conflicts rather than on interference and discussions on moral goodness. Seeing the child's outpourings as a kind of pressure or charge that he uses in order to gain strength of self and future decision making, we stand with the child learning how to steer this self-propelled entity. These are not feelings that surge up and must be tamed. We aren't talking about good, bad, and the right: We are standing in that good, bad, and right and helping the child arrive there intact. We are the guides rather than the determinants of the child's own organization of feelings. The child arrives at his perception of himself as a worthy person, primarily through intangible family dynamics and the quality of personal attitudes in daily living, rather than through teaching *about* beliefs (Macnamara, 2016).

Truly, in order to aggress, to drive one's growth into this state of wholeness from which a distinct individual person takes over, the child needs to preserve the old or earlier child-dependent states, and at the very same time begin to release the parent as the caretaker and carrier of this self-identity. This is what individuation is all about, really: becoming *me* while being separately curious about *you* (an outside-of-me entity). Being curious and wanting to know, becoming a best friend and then a partner and long-time intimate other that I always feel safe enough to say inside myself, "Just who are you, because you're sure not-me!" Once organized, reciprocal states are the skeletal strength of ongoing intimacy and mutual trust.

These little people, if they have been housed within the greater caretaking of a healthy adult, will still be a bit jittery, a bit easily excited over the small miracles of the day. Their imaginations are still firing away, linking one emotion-based fact with another and returning a quirky response back to us. They are willing to learn much faster than an older child's brain may want to because the imaginings from that wide-angle vision have not been narrowed. The essential question becomes how we respect and nurture this wider view and curiosity while children take on board more procedural tasks.

Of development, let us give ourselves a directive: to take our children and their mesmerizing growth—which moves forward and back, in and out—seriously, yet not literally. As Johnny said long ago, "I really just know everything already. I just don't have time to tell you it all. I haven't really learned that much."

CHAPTER 4

Zack and "The Usman" - Back to the Beginnings

Zack begins his work coming to each session dressed in complete Batman attire, including the mask and several odd tools on a belt. His cape and his mask seem to be the most important to him. He is obsessed with Batman and with all the parts that made him uniquely Batman. He carries a miniature toy of Batman, maybe 3-inches tall, in his hand. According to Mom, he sleeps in Batman pajamas. This obsessive need feels like a necessary and serious "disguise" to me; it is simply too early on for me to see into Zack's wounds. The disguise may also protect him against feelings of helplessness, like a second skin or shell.

Zack helped me to appreciate the prerequisite developments for becoming a self. What he worked hard on in therapy was an earlier developmental phase that had not taken hold for him. That dance of dependence/separation that builds trust in the self and then in the world had little trial-and-error rehearsals to count on. At 3½ years old, he was already being called to rely on skills for which little mapping existed, and what did exist seemed very worrisome. Zack led me back to that underdeveloped arena through his play. What I came to understand was after the fact, after Zack's process was already far along. In witnessing preverbal work, we are left putting our thoughts onto paper in hindsight, after the child has traveled some distance. As we trust the child's work, we are more able to endure this postponement of reason. In the meanwhile, I felt the growing reliability between us.

In understanding development, a metaphor that may help is to think of a series of 8 oz glasses of water. In healthy, trusting development, during one phase the young child makes use of the full glass. The psyche hands him another 8 oz as the next window of development presents itself. Every developmental phase needs a full 8 oz of water. The developmental window of 9-18 months is concentrated on separation. When a child experiences neglect or abuse, 5 of the 8 oz goes to hanging onto any safety from the parent. Little is left for the development that presents itself during this time. The neglected child is able to offer 3 oz to building separation. The next window, of expressing "no" as often as possible in order to experience the power of being separate, already has a weakened capacity to practice that great word. He might make every effort to spend about 3 oz during this available dynamic. The degree of safety in an earlier developmental window plays a crucial role in whether or not it is okay to practice the power of a self. By the time this child enters preschool, interior developmental mapping is confusing. The child might attempt to stick up for himself when another child takes a toy, but all he has available is an earlier developmental effort of biting. So he uses that. Or he senses that other children are moving more confidently than he can, and he goes quiet. Zack chose this option.

It is so important to understand how vital early developmental windows automatically open and close, pushing the child forward from the interior, to challenge himself in relationships that grow increasing complex. Zack was already suffering relational, trusting, vulnerabilities when he entered his preschool setting. In some ways his intellectual development continued to push him forward. While learning the give and take of peers, he was suffering from an increasingly vulnerable skill gap.

The Development in the Safety of Self

Zack will help us to understand what occurs when lack of safety hinders important infant developmental steps. His feelings remained disorganized because his environment was constantly and unpredictably unsafe. Zack used the freeze defense, which is simply playing dead. It is used when an animal sees there is no chance of escape or of surviving the attack. The freezing response includes abrupt motor and vocal restraint. Freezing in the context of an attack seems questionable. However, sudden immobility may automatically occur when one perceives little immediate chance of escaping or winning a fight.

Zack simultaneously remained as emotionally connected as possible to Mom, bypassing that developmental phase. Separation for him was, in the beginning, plainly difficult. He seemed closer to being 2 years old rather than his 3½-year-old self. Although my training alerted me to the possibility of domestic violence, I would learn about that near the end of our time together. Zack's vigilance that I first noted would make sense later. I heard about the hardships that his mother faced, and that Zack experienced, about 4 months into our work together. Remaining so deeply attached to Mom was a requirement because he depended on her fight – flight-flee instincts to register his own safety. Zack had thoroughly tucked his own sense of safety into his mother's efforts at safety, as if the two of them were in a constant and unpredictable storm that might take away necessary things in its wake. In keeping this tucked-in emotional position, Zack sacrificed movement toward some separation of self and future interdependent confidence. One core problem was that this solution of sorts could not remain in place. Zack's older sister by nearly two years had evidently not experienced some of the dynamics that burdened Zack.

Our developmental progress is an internal drive and cannot be waylaid for long. Development is an action and its force will continue, superseding crucial defenses. Its windows of change open and close - a deep, nearly involuntary sort of breathing mechanism in the psyche. What happens over time, if aspects of a given open window do not take place or partially take place, is a buildup of unfinished business. Zack remained in a very young dynamic of fused space in order to vigilantly track the immediacy of safety versus danger. Internal development moved on to next requirements along with missing pieces of his puzzle. His intelligence, for instance, continued to collect information from his environments, such as learning the alphabet and the phonetics of some words. But there was little-to-no motivation in revealing his intelligence because that potential energy was going towards maintaining instinctual alertness of danger. And letting others know what Zack was learning would make him more visible, undisguised.

By the time Zack entered pre-school, the next organic developmental windows of social learning were more than he could manage. His silence, acute stuttering when he tried to speak, and refusal to play with other children became noticeable behaviors. The missing pieces of separation and confidence festered in what we know as anxiety and depression, as if someone in there continued to ask, "But what about that trust section that got left out?" "What about the esteem it takes to show up in the class of kids and hold my own? I can't, most days." And Zack couldn't, any day.

Zack was building a secondary defended self that would keep his growing and vulnerable ego in some kind of supposed safety. Over time, unchecked, this imaginary quality would become more dominant and rigid, and his authentic self would need to take second place behind a false sense of safety. Zack might have continued to remain more in a world of his own making, unwilling to broadcast his real self. In children this often parallels the symptomatic behaviors of autistic traits in its disconnections. Unknown to anyone at the time, Zack was dipping into a strong innate intelligence in order to maintain a sense of safety. Over time, too, Zack would likely have bartered connection with others for his own perceptions of safety. When the psyche must choose, it will commit itself to safety of the person at cost to relationship.

In the private pre-school he was enrolled in, his teachers were worried about his unwillingness to socialize with other children. When he did speak, Zack stuttered badly and was difficult to understand. However, his ability to be almost poetic, when he landed in real time and place, was tremendous. An example: I sometimes picked up Zack when he would otherwise have missed that week. Once we were traveling along, and Zack quietly ruminated that "the birds and the trees are both flying through the sky." These windows into language had no stuttering, which offered clues to Zack's internal world. He was fully present. Connection between himself and others, however, carried its edge and its uncertainty.

"Usman" Carrying the Relationship in Image

Zack's work was that of securing mutual interactive trust. This meant that he needed to go back to his original experiences of relationship. Given enough "muscle," he would then initiate building a safe and separate self. His process took place in the interior world of an "us" which was held in the image forms of two Batmen. Using Batman as his overarching image and vehicle of work, the Batman he brought from home primarily represented him. This Batman was a developmental being, growing toward some power and reflection. Batman carried the heroic work of becoming human and embodied. The second Batman, who lived in the playroom's collection, carried Zack's transformative work. Zack immediately called him "Usman." *Us*man carried the meaning of the primal trust of infancy, where he still lacked enough assurance. At the time, Usman wasn't merely a representation, but was very much alive with the meanings this little toy carried. Usman *was* us. I was assigned a surrogate location in his play, a full-on participant so that together we might update Zack's own sense of self. For a period of time, Zack and I merged into this *us*, which had been too threatened during the growth of his infant self. In that threat, development had stalled out. Usman sustained the changes that I would carry with Zack until he could shoulder them himself. His healing was accomplished through the unlanguaged play of sand and miniatures that create worlds of relationships. Relationships in this modality of play are more metaphoric and symbolic and less in need of conversation. Usman carried the story of mending. Zack himself narrated this powerful approach in his story through the toys that became alive.

Every week Zack scanned my presence for a false and dangerous domination, and not finding it, went about his work. When he came into the playroom, there was a quietness between us during which I felt Zack's own vigilance focused on me. Was I a safe person? Zack couldn't manage eye contact. His halting speech told me that he needed my presence, not my words. It often felt as though words from thinking spaces were like stones that splashed into his work with their disturbances. These are the indicators the therapist watches for in order to weigh in on the child's readiness to seek attachment. Now and again I attempted to find an island of thought, but Zack's body would tense, exhibiting a withdrawal from this united space we found ourselves in. Or he might throw a toy angrily into the wet, splashing me. In early moments of finding one another, I felt the flooding I created when Zack literally jumped away from me or wet his pants. Intrusion seemed to occur when I asked him about how his week had gone or commented on the danger I saw between two toys in the tray. Even naming that he had hung his cloak on the hook could interrupt his silent need to put us both, immediately, into the images of the two Batmen. Usman needed to be alive as soon as we were alone together in the playroom. I learned to understand his efforts to remain in a preverbal space where most of his first 5 months of therapy time occurred. As he consistently seemed to find me present for him, he slowly left his disguise on the coat hook. In this, he recovered and repaired trust and then went on to construct a safe enough sense of self. All this was done with very little talk between us of what he might do that day, what had happened in his own environment, or where we were heading. Now and again Zack let me know what meaning had just stepped into the play by narrating Batman's and Usman's realities.

The us-ness of Usman was to be the vehicle that would convey Zack first back into deeply unfinished developmental separation and then forward, through intense anxiety, toward a self-identity that would speak out loud. So, Usman, one might say, represented the "us" prior to a "him," the profound need to be sheltered within an "other" in order to confidently hatch into a "me." This "us" represented a developmental need prior to the age of 1. To distinguish a self apart from Mom's ongoing efforts to find safety seemed an overwhelming task. But I didn't know this when we met. What I saw was a very small masked Batman.

Before we imagine a new self with Zack, we might look at what that word *self* directs us to. To illumine "self": "the total, essential, or particular being of a person: the individual" and "the essential qualities distinguishing one person from another." In its root, s(w)e-, this small word holds deeply ingrained images: "one's own; prince; created from oneself." Who would imagine Batman, or Usman, for that matter, to be a prince! Zack had yet to imagine himself as princely, as worthy of standing alone in his creation of self.

Batman and the Use of the Hero

Zack's early work involved establishing safety for Batman. He created the image of a boy building tinfoil wings and becoming kin to Batman. Batman would be able to do the difficult work that Zack's self was still far too immature and unnamed to do. This tinfoil-winged-Robin character prepared the way for the Usman that would take on the weight and power of a new safe relationship. Later on, he would again try being a boy, unmasked and capable. First things first, however. As Zack worked away at this tinfoil-enveloped boy, his own cape that he wore got hung inside the room. The cape moved from being a part of his own concrete disguise to being in the tray as an image. This is not to say his own cape entered the tray. Zack was laying his own vulnerabilities into symbols where they would be safe to construct a new protection before trying this newness on out in the world.

Usman, the Zack-and-therapist shared feeling state which now held itself together in a living space, became more and more ill each session as Zack's anxiety and anger increased. The images and their feelings were pulling out feelings, like any good poultice, that had chronically overwhelmed Zack. Sometimes I felt confused over who was Batman and who was Usman. I still feel that confusion when I read my old notes. I still truly believe we must take the risk of getting lost in order to go to the wordlessness of the very young child, having been trained to hold the unknown without truly becoming lost. Our risk reveals that we understand, so that the child, feeling seen, can approach a new level of trust. Stepping into that space gives us the embodied understanding of what it really takes for the child to build trust and be willing to be found. After all, taking the risk of being lost and truly being lost are quite different. At the same time, the risk of unsure footing puts us far closer to the child's efforts to be found.

This entire dance, of being within the child's felt realities while sustaining some semblance of separateness, is the dance of transference. Transference is the quality of permeability of the therapist's mind, the willingness to receive the child's raw material and attend to that child's self. Empathy results from this right-brain-to-right-brain attunement. The confusion around transference is often that therapists surrender their thinking. This isn't true. Receptivity in the emotional, heart-felt spaces in a human being do not scrap one's ability to observe and think. The heart, a priority in transference, has a great capacity to think. Felt understanding transfers easily to mutual understanding when we have done our own work and can remain in this permeable space together with the child and the child's need. What we often experience is confusion as our own right brain acclimates to the implicit perceptions from the child's self. Our own shadowy material may surface in these shared spaces.

When he is able to express feelings through these powerful characters, there is no stutter at all. As he moves deeper into his feelings, Zack brings babies into his play. Nervously he states to me, "The bad guy said, 'You can't save yourself, Batman!' But the Batman did save his self. If a child got dropped in the sewer, Batman could really save him. He could. His cape gets icky stuff on it. A little child is in the sewer. He is tied up in a chair in the sewer. He needs to yell for help." (Zack tells me to holler for help now. I give voice for a "bad boy" whose punishment is sewer-sitting.) The images and feelings of a sewer, being helplessly in it, tied to it, sicken me.

During this time together, Zack produced images that felt alive and that sometimes drained me of my thoughts. Large bugs came toward babies, crawling out of steaming volcanoes. The babies tried to find shelter and failed. In a large castle, the Grim Reaper closely followed Zack's Batman, silently hitting Batman when he got close enough. This process, which reveals great fear and a lack of safety, needed to be held and expressed. And at the end of a tough session, I attempted some comment on Batman's true strength working this helplessness out. As those first raw feelings safely surfaced and were understood and contained, Zack progressed in development, using his toy representatives to begin the work of separation. Two challenges located themselves in these expressions of anxiety. One was Zack's experiences in an unsafe environment. The second one was that Zack himself was stretching toward a separation that he would need to master, urged on by intrinsic developmental demands. This meant that he would need to experience a personal self that became stronger as he moved away from his mother's protective filters.

Zack began hanging more and more of his costume, one piece at a time, on a hook inside the therapy room. He was full of questions about the toys, and why was Batman in here, anyway? Then he would return to his work theme. I am not certain he wanted answers or responses to his questions. It was as if we were efficiently passing through that developmental phase of "babbling" during which a parent is at hand to mirror back the sounds themselves as meaningful and joyful. Zack needed my enjoyment of him, while I attended to the growing announcements of his realities in the tray.

Batman is now dying. The Grim Reaper had struck him in the heart. "It's his power. It's where his heart is." Later on, the Grim Reaper fatally hurts Usman, who must go to bed. Meanwhile, Zack could now tolerate having no personal disguise. He comes in his little-boy self, at times hanging a cape or a mask on the hook, as if to honor the placeholder of Usman.

Story in Image Form

The images were now carrying Zack's story. We wove back and forth, in and out, between the toys he chose and the meanings of the images. What happened to Batman and Usman was Zack's story unfolding in its metaphoric language. The image of Usman held very real harm being done. Zack was too young to tell me "My father hurts me." But he was able to let me know that Usman's heart had been struck and that it was very important that

I saw this event in his story. He knew I had seen Usman getting hurt. Being seen with a hurt heart had not harmed Zack himself. Zack trusted that I gave credit to who Usman was that I was a part of this adaptation from Batman to Usman. Perhaps Zack's own cape became the armor that had defended Usman and Batman. As Zack trusted that somehow he and I would make it through whatever it was that was coming alive in these images, he could hang up his own cape. And in the tray, Batman simultaneously shed his armor.

Usman and Batman then begin an odd imaginal journey of two becoming one Batman. Usman dies, in part because he cannot see and simultaneously must see better; his hurt must be covered. Zack covers the eyes with a band-aid. Zack's metaphor tells me that before, he, an individual, would not be visible. To be so was dangerous. The danger had forestalled speaking up and building a language of "me" and "I." At home he has his mother cut off the mask to his cloth disguise. In the next session, Zack states clearly, "Momma said not to take off Batman's head. But I can scratch off the mask, and there'd be a boy underneath. He could see." Authentic. What we have here is a quiet and thorough integration of the pre-one-year-old development: the mother remains attuned while the baby learns "to see," to look through the eyes of a me that can tolerate a you becoming outside of who I am. Usman's blindness is being attended to, and as we attend, Zack inhales courage to allow the representative Usman to become one self: Batman. Momma cares for the representative, and it is Zack who steps onto less firm ground and creates the original truth from his momma's containment: that there would be a boy underneath. It's as if Zack says, "I think I'm inside the Batman outfit. I AM."

Another significant process also occurred here. As trauma takes root within the young child, imagination is less and less safe. To believe that what the child imagines makes sense, the child must have an exterior other that holds and brings about the authenticity of the what-if world. Without this, imagined play loses its juiciness and potency for creating a symbolic world. It becomes concrete, edgy, and too hard. Children who carry trauma sometimes do not know how to play when we first introduce them to the playroom and the toys. They have landed in a world in which imagining has not been attended to. To adapt to the parent in order to not be hurt, playing becomes frivolous. In staying with Zack's own belief in Batman, Zack's mother had agreed with Zack's need to help Batman see, without having to cut off his masked head. She understood that his play held deep seriousness and she didn't challenge what he needed. Zack accepted this new view of his difficult play. His need to navigate *seeing* remained safely in its image, while momma navigated Zack's anxious efforts to take off Batman's mask while he took off his own.

In another session, Zack takes a staff, and one by one strikes Batman's muscles, stating, "There. Now Batman's human." But at home, when he asks his father for help with these significant toys, he is thoroughly and harshly discounted. Zack comes to the next session quietly. He tells me about this event. His comment is "I want you to find me a Popeye who eats spinach and gets strong. I have spinach in my pockets for when I need it [strength]." This is the first time Zack verbalizes a personal experience from home. He is strong enough to feel the difference between his felt comprehensions and his father's unwillingness to support him.

It is difficult to peer into Zack's evolving narration without feeling the sadness in his story. What becomes so vital is that he himself is organizing his worry and pain into a narration that, through these miniatures, someone else is witnessing. Someone else carries the burden with him. He has named that someone Usman.

Zack again takes the smallest babies, puts them next to the volcano, away from large threatening bugs. He continues with the event: "Batman takes his cape off. He knows who he really is.

Zack and "The Usman"- Back to the Beginnings

The bad guy thinks Batman isn't really Batman. He thinks he's pretend. But he's not." The metaphoric work mirrors Zack's own landscape now.

"Batman is lifting barbells to get strong."

A child's imagination is serious work, and in need of protection by caring adults. Zack, now age 4, had the strength to lift a threatening shadow away from his own budding self, and to begin calling out his own name: someone who can turn toward this inner process that strengthens individual personhood. Images that Zack had enlivened were organizing indigestible material into creatively new attitudes. While severe anxiety continued to threaten this newly found recognition, his use of play kept his development moving forward.

After this, I heard the details about the constant abuse in the home. Mom decided to move back to her support system, across states. Zack was frightened about this move. I ask what we might do to use his power to move. His response: "I got to make a house." He pours all of Batman's things—cape, belt, staff—into the tray. He draws a circle in the wet sand. "What can we use? What do we need?" he asks out loud. "Make a big 'Z' so we can make a house. A big house. What can we use? We're supposed to see what we need." Here is the great metaphor of Sight. He is frustrated, and so am I. He begins putting in large blocks of wood, like monoliths. Is this struggling house-image an effort to have something, a self-created transitional image from our work, to push forward into the unknown?

One possible meaning to this building effort is that Zack was risking so much in order to confront a concrete upcoming reality, of flying in an airplane to a new home that had no images in his internal map. He would need to traverse his imaginary capabilities with a very concrete world. This thrusts him into sort of "walking the walk," not remaining in a younger state of this "us" world. The house he attempts reminds me of a turtle making thorough use of the house on his own back. Except Zack isn't sure that there's any safety if he lands in a 3-D landscape without somewhere to crawl into.

Zack picks up Batman, who now needs new armor. He creates his own new protection over Batman, made of foil. (Recall his first efforts to introduce a relationship between Batman and a human boy by creating wings of foil.) The eyes are not covered, as they need to "see." The armor needs to have an open space over Batman's "heart," the bat emblem. With Batman now watching and aware by the side of this creation, he continues on with the house. He fashions the walls with his hands, telling me that "I think and think about protection and come up with nothing. Nothing works." We continue to discuss his need for safety, which in our talk is directed at major changes. He is, however, also addressing his general sense of helplessness and the fears he experiences at home. Slowly he comes to realize that his protection might involve "only my choice..." I say yes. "Then this house has no windows. People can't see in." He puts a lid over his house and tells me to take care of this house when he leaves.

Zack had earned, through his own bravery, the power to choose when to see and be seen. He could open the windows, and close them when danger came close. The dignity in this "only my choice" is that Zack could begin to trust his own instinctual sense of safety now. Developmentally, Zack had returned to a much younger self to launch a separate self. This self would have more say in his safety and would need to build stronger trust in his own instincts.

Zack's Batman outfit had acted as a layer of skin of which he otherwise had too little. Zack was unusually intelligent. Intelligence and its sensitivities do not weather well in an environment of abuse. The young child dips into key traits within and begins constructing disguises and masks that are really too heavy to wear over an ego that is not yet organized to know any difference. The disguise will take on a "false front." Winnicott calls it the false self (Winnicott, 1971). The false self is an artificial sense of self that people create very early in life to protect themselves from re-experiencing trauma and shock in intimate relationships.

Intelligence seems to work hard to pull a person away from chaos. Zack had created an image that his imagination held onto very tightly. His intelligence had engaged to the point where speaking in real time was challenged, and being among other children seemed exhausting to him. A false self was not yet stable, but in another window of time, he could have built enough strength there so as to become intolerant of his own vulnerabilities. Batman was still hanging in there, an imaginative connection with a superhero.

Usman was an entity that seemed to pop up like a transitional object: that which is neither real nor unreal, but a symbol that holds the merged space. Because Zack *was* in a paradox that was growing thinner: being both tucked under his mom's safety and slowly (through developmental growth) realizing that this was not a safe option, either. In this, he took me in and, judging enough safety, returned to a much younger developmental arena of shared unity in order to try again. It is like a pole vaulter who, in order to clear the jump, must step back far enough to strengthen the leap across. Seeing the transitional object as a leap into a transitional space, Winnicott states, "It is not the object, of course [Usman, in this case], that is transitional. The object represents the infant's own transition from a state of being merged with the mother to a state of being in relation to the mother as something separate" (Winnicott, 1971).

Usman entered as the form that could carry Zack backward into unfinished separation in order to leap forward into the trust required to truly construct an internal hero. Batman had been his mask, behind which as Zack said, "There would be a little boy." The fantasy hero, sickened and having lost his sight, began to move aside enough for the "us" merged self to find its footing and reveal a self that felt and acted upon its Zack-ism. Usman held the pieces together in order that Zack could uncloak the little boy. We might say that Zack remained within a shell of a hero and then hatched again, as a little-boy self. I could only have faith that this move would further solidify a home in his little body. Those trappings, the bits and pieces that had formed a sense of self-definition, were left in my care as the witness to a Batman who, as Popeye, had a big task ahead.

His work was unfinished when he, his sister, and his mom moved away. But during the time he had been coming, while his disguise fell away, Zack had risked social play at his pre-school. He had become quite popular because of his unusual capacity to articulate play and imagination. At age 4, he also knew how to read simple books, and much to the surprise of the teachers, could sit with others his age and entertain them with reading some real words. There was no stuttering. I believe Zack came in as Batman and created Usman as the transitional symbol of a trustworthy relationship, working hard to transform helplessness into something human and doable. He left as Zack, with the image of Popeye, working to be a strong and rather organic hero that had his own body's muscles and his own embodied and righteous anger to power up and then internalize a real boy.

CHAPTER 5

Orion: Implicit Memory

I recall a young child who, by age 4, had been moved three times in foster care. She invented a game of rushing toward me to be caught because there was a monster chasing her. We did this two or three times in one session. In the next session she played this game again. The first two times she flung herself on me, I felt a lifelessness which worried me. I held both this deadness and her anxiety as she ran toward me again. I watched her face as she crossed the small distance. Her body seemed to take on a terror, so that I nearly wanted to look for the monster myself. As she grabbed me, her body was visibly shaking, and her eyes were huge. The monster had become real. So had the trust she had hoped to rely on me to maintain. We had aligned, right brain to right brain. Within the charge of these two polarities, her somatic memory joined with her affective memory, and here came the monsters, charging into the now. The work immediately following this recovery was difficult, and it often regressed into much younger states of being. At the same time, this child became more able to cross the distance between her well-defended self, toward the trusting heart of an adoptive parent. This adult is poetic, imaginative, and vulnerable.

So this is where we therapists enter, in the profound core need of a child to be remembered. To be remembered approaches the great need of being known, being cared for by someone whose care makes us real. Remembering also includes developmental pieces that have been darkened out so that they remain unseen. They do, however, speak loudly, sometimes roaring their presence.

One crucial place where play therapy heals is in the realm of memory. We will need to temporarily loosen up our linear comprehensions to navigate the child's own subjective use of remembering and implicit realness. This trust is unconditionally given by the child, wrapped as it is in the requirement of that great word: Dependency. Having no doubt in us, we are asked to let go of presuppositions and play: play together, co-create, be serious within the finding of each other.

Parent as Regulator

Perhaps a little confusingly, the regulating adult serves as a filter located outside the being of the young person: the vital other who is literally an other. As children develop, the essential and safe adult is the outer parameter of the child's self, remaining in place as a guide and filtering system. Think of this, perhaps, as the child's second skin. The parent's regulating envelope orchestrates incoming experiences with the child's ongoing capacity to absorb those inputs. The parent ruminates on the child's temperament and past experiences as well as the present—hunger, tiredness, and current stamina. How each child blends imagination and emotion, toward an interior stability that will be known to the child simply as "me," requires this envelope. Through these outer parameters of attuned care from the parent(s), the child will eventually find himself at home, that is to say *his* home within his body as his personal skin holds the shape and confidence of a self.

The parent's essential task is to safeguard and synchronize the child's engagement with the intensities of outer reality while the child builds an inner identity. As this "me" gradually becomes firm enough, the parent mentors the child into the thrills and burdens and responsibilities of the human landscape. It is as though the parent's thorough engagement of the child's developing self allows growing trust to become owned by the child over time. And it is the interior conviction of the parent's attuned care–that "you matter to me"–which promotes the child's capacity to become an individual.

That safe adult is, within the child's sense of self, simultaneously acting upon the requirements for protection and oversight in the child's development of a confident identity. Step back into Zack's work a moment. Zack's outer shields were not working: one shield-carrier was brittle with violent-feeling responses and the other remained vigilant in his attempts to sustain safety. Zack lacked the motivation or incentive to reveal his needs and his meanings. To do so was dangerous since random efforts to speak up in one way or another did not necessarily work for him. Take, for example, his request to see Batman's eyes, which resulted in a harmed Batman. Zack's presentation was one of a shut down 3-year-old, a child who stuttered heavily, and hardly engaged with anyone. He was becoming preoccupied with building his own shield of Batman as the armor he needed. That fantasy would not have met his real human need to be seen and heard and understood. It is hard to know who this young highly intelligent child could have become had Batman continued to stand in as that second skin. In his work, it became clear that Zack was carving out a silent world inside of which a little boy did lots of "sewer-sitting."

Zack used Batman to represent a vulnerable entity who accepted the burden of a hero who would need to become very sick and blind. At a felt level, he provided "Usman," Batman's otherness that was a new effort for Zack, with the task of going on the journey into relationship. "Us" blindly traveled into a hurt place, together picking up what we could, shifting that big old neurology whose primary charting came from the injured lives of his parents, into some new landscape that he decided was "only my choice." And he held on to his integrity after his dad thoroughly shamed Zack's belief that if he "scratched off the mask, there'd be a boy underneath." That had been the psychic space he was hunting for in this process, and he found it, and in finding himself there, Zack initiated building his own second skin through relationship and attachment. He would have to work hard, even changing hero-images to Popeye, if he was to build some protection round this newfound self. Recall the anxiety of building his last image: the house with no windows. Even though heavily shuttered, this house was a very real second skin, a dwelling place where his last commitment was to give his process over to me to watch, to continue to "see." In this image, Zack let me know that he was not yet strong enough to claim a confident self. But he had moved his meaning-maker to a more authentically connected space. Zack's work unveils the urgency with which our children approach being found, and the need to state clearly that in creating "only my choice," the safety of a separate self manifests.

Memory as Stored Up Feeling States

Memory can be referred to as the vehicle in which we store our experiences. Storage occurs through sensations, through our senses of the world and of the people around us. Implicit memory takes in the felt environments through all of our senses. All of that non-verbal meaning creates its own map. Little people are authoring their days, moment by moment. And implicit memory is taping those moments, interlacing meanings and feelings and body responses into a "this is me" identity. This is implicit reality. When we offer tools like art and sandplay, and we offer ourselves as the access port to a shared understanding that will reveal itself in the play of the moment, it is as if we are in the past-present. Implicit memory has opened up, coming into the moment here and now, and letting us peer into the map that this particular child has created from the scratch and sniff of experience. Memory updates as a map that considers and includes new information as it is experienced. Because a child's ego is not separate enough to sustain its own containable history, memory refreshes itself to keep up with its task of growth.

When working with children, even memory, ultimately, must be addressed from a perspective that is not fully defined. When we piece together the child's still-indefinite time awareness with memory that is still available to update its meaning, all these pieces together braid into a very forgiving memory. In a play arena of relational trust, this elasticity works in favor of healing. The child's play steps into a combined sensation of trust and thus the willingness to show us his own experiences. Sequestered experiences and their meanings are revealed in the play. Affects of the current experiences merge with the affective experiences of the past. What we see and hear are sometimes confusing bits of past experience blended with current experience. What we are really seeing is a full-bodied, affect-ridden map whose effort is to keep track of this particular child and the ways he understands his days.

Those past experiences are still available to a person whose defenses are not fully formed. The child uses play to embody her meanings of experiences. Her behaviors, which may not be working at all for her in her environments, enter the play, charged with current experiences and a memory of recent past experiences with their subjective meanings. Behaviors are so important to approach with compassion, as behaviors are the exterior consequence of what we might call somatic memory. Memory located in the body and kept in an unaware state are highly likely to erupt, to act outwardly, when the meanings of the somatic memory impinges on the event right now. Unaware overwhelming feelings from a past experience and the current trigger collide. Overload of this past and present will inevitably call for our help through an onrush of behaviors.

Recall that babies comprehend attunement and therefore safety through their five senses and the skin. This is the earliest and most primitive charting on one's own internal map: the safety of the other who in the first few months is still "us." When current trust is disrupted, that earliest most primitive mapping is where the child goes. Our children will make use of primal and on-hand communicators, their bodies and their behaviors, when these collisions occur. The fact is, they simply do not have the mental language to tell us what went wrong while it went wrong. A constant failing on our adult parts occurs when we believe that a young child can tell us in words when the use of words in the brain is just not on-line yet.

As early as 3 years old, some children are able to bring some language to their breakthrough behaviors only after they feel safely attuned with a safe adult. That is when you hear, "I don't know how to make my hitting stop, Mama. It happens," or "I can't get the food down my throat. My throat doesn't work" or "There's too much noise. Even the radiator makes noise, and those lights do, too." These are not comments made when an adult asserts, "Use your words!" Before a child can make use of words, the parent will have needed to mentor a palette of emotionally-based words that have been linked to the available experience. Practice needs to have occurred involving a calm adult brain with which the child can remain linked.

Memory enters as vital, and at the same time, unstable. As these recent meanings and linked current experiences are brought into the room in miniature play-representatives or puppets or drawings, the child's access to her neurology in the body also connects. It is crucial that the dynamic trust in the relationship contains the child's intensifying outbreaks of unconscious but triggered right-brain (meaning-making) nervous system experiences.

Relationship and Memory

Memory is full of feeling. Feelings, embedded in memory, are where the treasures of meaning lie. When we hear adults say they do not remember their childhoods, we may be looking at their histories as having not been attended to fully in their own times and events. When we can't remember, we have also lost a degree of meaning to what it was we passed through. Although at one time we were fully alive as children, the relationships between the adults and ourselves were compromised by partial attention, the "Mmm-hmm" of accepting a child's babble without full attention and acceptance of the effort the child made in making meaning through shared space.

Memory rests in the fullness of being understood in relationship. And clearly, being understood carries the dynamics between two people. The therapist and the child stand in this liminal space, and with the capacity we call relating, create an affect that approaches that of the parent. Relationship and trust are held and stabilized, and then returned to the child's self with compassion. This cycle, of going outward to another, being recognized, and then returning with a feeling of "You heard me; I am that important," assures memory that identifies "I am safe. You know me. You love me."

Child psychology often talks about pre-verbal experiences. In this a priori world, the child's meaning is based on a hypothesis rather than an experience. And yet, our culture, with its bent on the intellect, often requires a systematic and scientifically based set of experiments to verify knowledge. Child development has been able to establish a backbone of fact from a history of infant/caregiver interactions. At all times, research-based understanding must include the child's own knowledge resources and how we might listen for the child's communications. It is clearly not that the child does not remember. The child's memory may constantly be brimming with feeling-based memory, a private knowledge of one's experiences. But that memory developmentally lacks oral language for this form of communication.

To truly give the child's internal world, with its fast-growing personhood, the merit it deserves, we need to step further, beyond scientifically based experiments. Children themselves have helped us understand their less-than-verbal worlds. While by ages 3 and 4, these worlds are not so much pre-verbal, they do continue to be pre-logical. Children's worlds, when held with intimate care, have not and need not be examined for objectivity. They do not yet belong in the objective environment of proof, but are safeguarded by a good-enough parent or therapist as containing and revealing the meaning the child has made of her experiences.

A friend of mine has an almost 4-year-old son. This adult friend lost her father suddenly before her child was 2 years old. Orion was very close to his grandfather, who was a favorite playmate with this imaginative little one. It was difficult to figure out how to explain that Orion would be unable to visit his grandpa. Orion's visits to his grandparents had been full of rituals and traditions: filling the birdfeeders, checking out the neighborhood meadows on walks, and playing music as a family group. These traditions were to become so important in linking Orion's implicit memories with his own ongoing efforts to comprehend this deep loss for everyone.

Orion's mom had gotten two photos of the last time they had all been at the beach, and she put them in Orion's room. Many months later, when Orion was closer to 3 years old, he brought one of the photos to his mom. "Grandpa," he points and says. His mom connects the trip to the beach, offering her son grounded remembering to his internal felt meanings of his grandfather. This is where adults support the child's internal meanings the most. Offering shared memories to Orion pulls implicit feeling states into a shared feeling state between mom and little boy. This activity stabilizes his own feelings, and furthers his ability to make sense of his loss.

Orion: Implicit Memory

"Grandpa take me to beach," Orion says. *"That's right,"* Mom responds. *"That is from when you went to the beach with Grandpa. Do you remember going to the beach with your Grandpa?"* Orion considers this. *"I not like the sand. Grandpa carry me. We find rocks."* Orion continues to study the photo. *"Grandpa loves me."*

Orion is deeply resonating, through his mom's efforts, to a current love between himself and his grandfather. Implicit memory is now active and useable: it is real, and the current of love is being held by Orion's mother for its safety and exploration

"Yes, sweetie. Grandpa loved you very much. You were his favorite little guy." *"Wanna see Grandpa,"* Orion states. This is his first time he had asked to see his grandpa in the nine or so months since his grandfather's death. Here is the space in which Orion's loss is now in the relationship between his mom and himself, with all of its potential meanings.

"I'm sorry, honey. We can't see Grandpa anymore. He died."
"He die?"
"Yes."
"He come back?"
"No, honey. When someone dies, they can't come back."
"Why?"

This is as far as the two go that day. Later on, Orion continues to absorb this primary loss in his own ways, his parents watching over him and offering the links that say that they share this loss, and that they are there to affirm Orion's remembering. It is in this remembering of his grandfather that Orion is also remembered. He is linked to this profound love of someone he must move to an interior space. The shared traditions can now be made use of again and again. He has a song that his grandfather played with him, laughing and exploring the record as it played this song. Orion listens to that now. He has full ownership of the photos in his room. He might take them down and carry them about, and *sometimes slips them out of their frames in order to let the two of them travel together more easily.*

Recently, his family took a walk with Orion, to a meadow that held grandpa's favorite tree. Grandma shares the importance of this tree with Orion. Orion asks his family to pick a leaf so he could take it with him to put in his treasure box. This request on Orion's part is the consequence of a mother, a father, and a grandmother holding space for a very young child.

Later, while his grandma sits with him, Orion says that he wishes Grandpa would call him on the phone and if he could, would he come to visit. This is another moment of building memory and acceptance. Grandma says that Grandpa is somewhere that makes those things impossible and that she knows we are all sad and miss him. "If Grandpa is deeply sad about anything in this place where he is, it is that he cannot spend time with Orion because he loves him so much." Grandma shares some of her own ways of still being with Orion's grandpa. He listens very carefully and clarifies some bits. He checks Grandpa's photo that he carries. Slowly and completely, Orion is coming to understand the loss of such an important person. He will continue to revisit this place of relationship in his past, updating it while he integrates what love and loss mean to him.

The Child's Ways of Knowing

Now, nearing age 4, Orion knows what he needs from down in his bones. The memory of this important person is now a part of his own authorship. The adults in his life have walked with him through his seemingly random feelings and expressions, his sensations and his wonderings. Orion's memories, including many nonverbal markers, such as being carried when the beach sand was too intense, are now available. In the world of implicit memory and ongoing reality, young children will move forward as they internalize that they themselves are loved and this being loved remains accessible. When memories have remained safe, the child has added chapters in his life as references that can be accessed when called upon. We have found and have been found within our own story. We have located ourselves. We are able to go back as adults and find ourselves and the material that made us who we have become.

This is a difficult area to discuss. We attempt to comprehend through dissection, pinning down, and interpretation. That leaves us talking *about* rather than being open to what our children reveal. Orion's mom and dad did not interpret. This might have meant that they tell the story of what literally happened to Orion's grandfather. If they had, Orion's own perceptions would not have been well enough understood by any of them, most of all by Orion himself. They sustained a space in which Orion might come to terms, his terms, with this profound and sudden loss. Orion's implicit memory now carries him along in his relationship with his grandfather. His meanings have room to be refreshed and updated as he grows. This doesn't mean that Orion will someday relate a smooth story of this relationship. Shared memory as historic facts will be built by way of the braiding of stories his parents, grandmother, and others will tell. He will also have his story, his memory, of this great wizard of a grandfather. Orion's ability to internalize his relationship with his grandpa allows that relationship to be a life-long touchstone.

The articulation of implicit memory, and then implicit reality, occurs in play and attunement. It is the world of dreams, metaphor, and inspiration. That world carries in itself strong feelings and tones, which relate the subjective understanding of the child to us. Language will serve as the mediator, the dynamic that encodes one's own meaning-making, files it into a subjective me-ridden order, and builds a history from this authorship. We might say that each of us has our very own creation myth. Language is alive and stunning when we keep it in its subjective development, as the result of image-building rather than the verbal ability to communicate. This will hopefully assist us in crediting just how young children do communicate. Orion's adults continued to gather together the signals that Orion sent, not running ahead to steady his developing understanding. They might have intruded in his metaphoric and meaning-making expressions with their need to make sense. Sense-making and meaning-making are two different routes of discovery. An adult who longs to help the child make sense prematurely has intruded and betrayed the child's creation myth which continues to be written in the meaning-making self of the child.

We use the word "sanctum" in therapy to refer to the confidential container that we keep watch over and within as witnesses and therapists. We who commit to a space as free as possible from intrusion, a dedicated place waiting for the child's work, are responsible and responsive to this germane space in which trust and attunement hopefully take hold.

Bring to mind how Delilah demanded that I remember her bird museum, which held her own story of a past that had not been narrated. Memory is not a noun. It travels, dances, stops and shudders, laughs, takes photos with an interior lens that remembers. How might we talk about something that is always moving, digesting, hungry for more of that being seen in order to see-better?

The implicit perceptions in the right brain are pre-occupied with something truthful, something that is *me* and *mine* because of *us*. There is a standing room only for the two people who remain vulnerable to what is next, what is here. Implicit memory is a form and a consequence of recognition. What remains alive, living, in our remembering is the shared understanding, the space where two people stand and listen and assure that meaning happens through the course of the two.

Part II

Stages of Treatment in Play Therapy

CHAPTER 6

Eric and the Cat

I walked a little boy from his first-grade classroom every week. Before picking him up one particular week, his teacher let me know that this had been an unusually rough week, with classroom destruction that required putting other children out of the room for a period of time.

When I pick up Eric, he seems tenuously present. He is twitchy, so that even crossing the street at the crosswalk seems to upset him. As I offer my hand as guidance, I comment on his green sweater. He begins his own story. "The cat has green fur. She likes it that way. Oops! She's gone now! She just ran into those trees over there." Eric's use of metaphor tells me not to be direct. Following his cues, I say that her green fur helps to spot her and whoa! there she is! I could see her. Is she lost, does he think? "No. She knows we're watching. Her fur is really soft. Feel it." He stretches out his own green arm. I comment that I am glad to know that her fur is this soft and that she would stay warm until she feels safe enough to come with us.

I could have separated him from being the cat. Or, I could have assured the cat that we would be safe and that the cat could come with us. Both these options are not involved with Eric's efforts to find safety, something he does not feel at that moment. I would have been attempting to help him step out of his aroused

117

implicit memory and into his left, observing brain. I would have urged both of us to make more sense.

The Impact of Our Stories

We who work with children do so with an array of tools, models, theories, and our own belief systems. For many children, a good therapist is one who has done her or his own work, been trained in a broad enough range of skills, has a map of relational development, and is honest regarding her own limitations. In working with trauma, however, we are up against experiences that words can refuse to assist. Instead, we enter dynamics that the child carries as if they are his own story. But he himself is not located in that story. A child absorbs the effort to become who the parent defines as the child's self. When the parent has little self-awareness that would more readily contain his or her own past, the child inherits the parent's unconscious experiences, particularly those in the emotional realms. What has hurt the parent remains disorganized and susceptible to triggers from the child's own presence.

The Therapist as the Tool

Humbly, we ourselves are the best tool available. And sometimes the worst of the tools. In the end our relationship will attest to the core goodness of the child in our room. The effort to witness another's pain becomes less logical and more intentional, as does entering any landscape that has been sorely threatened. More often than not we must have built in ourselves the stamina to leave the known paths of therapy, knowing our way in the dark, to find the children who are literally and imaginally orphans.

This is not to say we go rogue. We are bound by ethics for a reason. The pathways can be difficult to witness and address in our youngest community members. And our training is essential to building and maintaining a critical, professional model that we live by. At all times, finally, we require other discerning professionals who are willing to hear our processes and those of our clients/patients. To see into the dark, we must check in, trusting the flashlights of clarity and observations from other professionals upon whom we can rely.

Children who have not found attached safety cannot tolerate sustained connections without more primitive and powerful feelings of danger emerging. Those primal feelings will apply pressure on adults for relief from these terrors. Fight, flight, and freeze activate. We face a child who is either absent from the relationship at hand or must act upon the pressure and find the relief of this pressure through destructive behaviors. The child seeks a return to calm in whatever ways possible, and this can often mean harming behaviors. The balm to disquiet is in relationship. This is where difficulties started and the return to those difficulties holds the repair.

Within about 10 minutes this separated cat aspect joins us, as Eric comments on having the cat follow us into the playroom. "Actually," he says, "she's just scared all the time. She's so shy, and then people think she can do stuff and she can't even hear 'em." I have so much more to go on, to help create places of safety for him. Eric had a set of parents who were severely addicted, and their ensuing behaviors were disorganized and violent. Eric had been removed only recently from this environment. He has no idea what to do, who to be, how to name his chaotic feelings. But the cat has some knowledge.

Following the cat, wondering together if she would get lost or would know her way through the woods with her green fur, brought me to Eric's interior gate. The toys that day were cats, and he was able to further define his pain. How would we make use of green fur, a cat running just beyond our reach, and a boy who could not hear classroom needs? How do we narrate all this and more into a diagnosis that then tells us which tool(s) to apply? We therapists may demand our own safety as we skitter into the woods of our words, compromising some required creative work in order to find the entryways into these children's lives who have stopped believing they can be found, yet are, of course, worthy of being found. Therapists will need a diverse set of tools. Understanding the deepest interactions required in infant development allows us to comprehend what a 6 or 7-year-old feels when safety and trust were constantly threatened. We must ask where is imagination in the lost maps of creating a self. And importantly, how are we ourselves to experience a child's defenses toward *not* being found, so that this child might feel our recognition of his pain and loss? We need to understand the implications each child reveals in play as we approach his potential state of loss and shame.

Therapeutic Road Signs

In our most at-risk children, there are unknown features in their interiors, with little language or history of common sense. We will find some features in the pockets of rage, in silence, in self-aggression, or other behaviors. The rage that Eric exhibited in his classroom pointed toward some unnamable feeling state that might claim him; might threaten his core (Kalsched, 1998). To experience such anxiety threatens the total annihilation of the human personality. This must be avoided at all costs and so, because such trauma often occurs in early infancy before any coherent ego is formed, a second line of defenses comes into play to prevent the "unthinkable from being experienced" (Kalsched, 1998).

One route toward understanding each human being's efforts to create and maintain an authentic self is to listen to each person's story. A child's authentic and original story has been tampered with when the environment has not felt and heard this child's

"Real." This authentic story within each child's self is the one that holds his essential gifts and existential truths that have yet to be spoken. The child conveys a wholly subjective self, and it is this innocence that preserves truths until such time as the child has grown to the place of thinking-about. Later on in healthy development, this child will both feel the subjective narration and listen for offerings and challenges from others.

Closer to the point is how this subjective landscape carries forward in development. Given a strong protective "skin" or filtering system of a parent, the child is allowed to absorb meaning and make more narrative of those meanings, without the impingement of others' internal beliefs. When the child grows from the inside to out, she is given the right to have her own story, and to make her own edits to that core. When her brain develops to include future reasoning and logic, she herself will develop the tools that enlist feel-to-think and think-to-feel dynamics. The crucial factor here is that the child must be nested in an adult's deep care. Relational care must be available and consistent. That care needs to model boundaries, forgiveness, generosity, while guiding the child's own curiosity of life moving forward. The safe relational environment that conserves the child's right of his origins story is pivotal.

Circling back, again to implicit memory and implicit reality, we can address how children create meaning. The therapist provides an attuned relationship that gathers a child's moments and holds them without tampering with them. This collecting process, in the heart of it, gathers in what trust the infant may have had. Play therapy will collect the scraps, and will make from them a safety net. All the while, the therapist sustains whatever trust the child grew within his first months of life. With this origin story ingredient in place, the child builds a renewing reality using feelings, body sensations, perceptions, and behavioral impulses.

Zack, who used Batman to reveal his own experiences, addressed so much in the imagery of the child in the sewer. That child became Robin, who became "Usman." And "Usman" embodied the wounded wholeness of Zack. This Batman would need to be very sick. His biggest ailment seemed to be that he could not see. His eyes were bandaged, and then he slowly became well again. Was Usman's blindness Zack's own suffering? What matters most is that Zack found his own path again, and with abuse still happening, he took on the image of Popeye. Zack had built enough stamina to address authentic and confusing feelings of anger and loyalty, and the experiences of a separate self.

The parent or therapist comprehends the child's own efforts to integrate a personal and subjective understanding of the child's own scrap collection. The greater the understanding offered, the broader the tolerance within the child for his own perceptions. This "trusting relationship would create an increased tolerance to 'be' with the myriad of feeling and body states that before may have felt too frightening, too overwhelming, to be taken into awareness" (Siegel, 2017). As windows of tolerance open wider, a child is far more able to attend to the other: to the teacher, the friend who is bossing on the playground, and, most importantly, to that internal instinctive voice that builds trust in one's self over time.

When the child feels safe, and is secured both to a trustworthy adult and to the interior instincts, implicit memory tumbles along writing the child's autobiography and meanings. The child's self-confidence in her interior narration will allow her to listen more closely to another's interpretation of her reality, without anxiety that she must constantly displace her knowing with another's. There is far less over-dubbing of one's reality upon another. Adult guidance is not the same as adult correction, but is rather the willingness to listen, witness, and wonder what options the child has presented from an ongoing implicit meaning-maker.

When that implicit voice is safe, the child's self is quite open to discussing a diversion from a black-and-white reality to a more curious and shared reality.

Curiosity is derived from the root word "to care, take care of, cure." Stretching on this a little, we might note that curiosity is a symptom of a return to health: the "desire to know or learn," the desire to authorize more of the world as meaningful to ourselves. It takes curiosity to maintain and expand on our origin story. When meaning has been integrated, we have made sense of what it was that drew us in. We have stretched a bit, taken in something new. In making sense, we will be able to narrate our perceptions to others. We have the capacity to build an argument based on our own truths and to adjust those truths when other truths impact us. We maintain balance in the relationship of interior self with conscious self, of someone deep in there with someone who is wondering about the landscape bringing information from there. When our own curious meaning-maker is congruent with the original stories we are packing about deep within, we have the joy of feeling "right with the world."

As the child develops, the urgency for a separate self grows. The child's own right-brain meaning-maker, the scribe to the child's experiences, wants more than understanding. Individualizing creates a need to understand the other and the outside components that are constantly affecting her own interior story. Her linkages toward another mirrors itself internally as she reaches inward to narrate her experience and its separateness from another's experience. This is the private rhythm of listening to the outside input, then listening to the inside, and finally discerning what of all this is hers to integrate.

When we tell children to "use your words," we will have needed to model over and over which kind of words we are talking about. We are most often referring to words that will speak their feelings and that will communicate to those outside of them what it is they want understood. Using language is the *result* of movement toward the left hemisphere of reason. It is not the result of simply having feelings. Too often our request or demand is that children skip a step in their own truths and simply tell us something from a list of feelings chosen by ourselves. When I asked a 4-year-old once what happened in therapy, he said, "I dunno. I'm supposed to talk about something, like 'feelings.' Then I get something to eat. That's it." When I talked with him about his weekly visits to a counselor, he said he did not like it because the chair was too big. My hunch was that he did not feel a connection with anything internally. There was nothing happening for him because nothing fit with his experience of himself.

Decoding the Communications of Memory

We are often struck with awe by the originalities that pipe up and into our more rational frameworks, and frustrated and grumpy when these human beings cannot listen or simply "cannot" whatever it is that is significant to us. Whether it is brushing teeth because it is time or lining up correctly for recess, these short members in our communities seem to have an interior conversation, or two or three, that at any given moment rules their responses to us. If we are not aligned, we move into reactionary spaces, and the child moves with us while still remaining connected with what seems "best" from their internal constructs. A small crack of trust suddenly becomes a chasm as we ourselves cease to guide and instead demand.

I worked with a little 5-year-old who had been permanently placed with her maternal grandparents. In kindergarten Maggie's behaviors were unpredictable. She might suddenly pick up her chair and throw it. At times Maggie covered her ears and began a loud steady hum. Or she might simply walk out of the classroom and into the principal's office to "use the phone." No one could make sense of what might suddenly cause Maggie to leave the room. She herself had no description for her behaviors. But, letting others approach her during these times might also fail. She and I started right there, in her need to run away. We walked from the school, around the outside of the building, over and over. Maggie might or might not want to bolt. I kept my own body between her and the street, ready to snap her up. But because I trusted that she knew my presence, she was able to practice hanging out with me. She might run ahead a bit, making my heart pound. But I stayed in my place, not chasing her, or calling her back. I used the image of a rubber band connecting our belly buttons, and when she went too far, my stomach hurt. After some ambivalence, she always returned. We were practicing her thinking and feeling what made her run rather than the two of us chasing down a feral animal. She accepted my interference, often returning to me jumpy and loud-voiced. All this was about building an alternate pathway to her impulsive survival reactions.

Maggie did not have adults in her life to help repair her instinctual survival care. Maggie's mom lived on the streets in another state. Her grandma had had her own traumatic upbringing as an immigrant who had often suffered homelessness. All these traumas influenced Maggie's own memories. Intergenerational trauma existed between all of her adult models. Maggie was separated from siblings who had been adopted and, as the oldest, whom she herself had cared for.

At one point Maggie had followed her cat into the street in front of her home. Her grandma had been livid, and called me to have a meeting with her and Maggie. The two were deeply triggered in their fear of danger and Maggie's own need to save the cat. Her grandma's triggers, she told me later, were of not being safe as a child while not helping her own parents find safety. When I attempted to make sense of this event, while both their triggers continued in the playroom, Maggie threw open the door and ran. I followed her to where she had wedged herself between a table and the wall. Her old fight-or-flight mechanism was clearly present. And I had seemingly joined with the grandma in the danger by my effort to think through the street situation. Maggie felt alone and betrayed by me. Slowly but surely, I coaxed her into my lap. After some time, she was able to say, "Everyone is gone now. I don't have nobody. I *had* to save my cat!" At least we had built enough trust that Maggie could make use of my presence and could forgive me for what she experienced as an ugly betrayal. Later she wrote the message, "I do want wen I grow up for a memrey uv you," meant to be given to her grandma. Maggie was able to tell her grandma that she did want to stay alive and not be hit by a car, or that she did want to not live in the streets like her own mother was doing.

What is a bit ironic is that those internal voices and maps the child is tracking are what we want to support unambiguously, since what is going on in there holds the child's own instinctive sense of safety, the ingredients to self-esteem and a personality that builds upon itself with assurance. Maggie's grandparents had told her to not go out into the street. To them, that was a fact. To Maggie, it was survival of the cat. Her cat held the only constant shared memory. When we adults demand that we be obeyed regardless of the faint voices continually offering substance to the child's behaviors, we are demanding that they override their own instincts. Those instincts watch over the child's own truths, and when an adult's grumpy self tells the child to hurry along our own paths of efficiency, adults compromise their trust in their truths. While we lecture about safety and obedience, we are simultaneously saying, "Listen to me because we both know *I am* safe. Follow my directives because I know what is best." While that may be true, we are training the child's neurologies to listen to someone who may not recognize her internal voice. We also tell her not to listen to someone who is a bad person. The conflict is this: adults might tell the child to listen to them simply because they are an adult, not because they understand the child's dilemma. At the same time that adult tells the child not to accept something from a stranger. If the child has not built an interior truth, there is little to comprehend the difference between these kinds of adults. Neither of the adults have heard from the child's own perceptions.

The emotional space to maintain is to hear the child's viewpoint while also maintaining an adult position of safety and clarity. In an ideal world, her grandparents would have first calmed themselves from their terror that something bad *could have* happened. Then they would have been more able to show Maggie how to stay safe even though the cat had made an unsafe choice. To Maggie, in that moment of running into the street, her triggers announced that she and the cat were one and the same. She was left to sort out who was bad, who was safe, and what to do if those hyper-alert instincts begin beeping again. Young children have a highly sensitive instinctual self, one that does not have language to support the information they are given from this interior. They do not have on board the more sophisticated discernments that might access reasoning. They are still inside the parent's filtering system. If that filter is faulty, children locate themselves in their own immature survival system. It will take even longer, once the child enters school, to reach through this internalized reactive linkage.

Behind the Power Struggle

There is an immediacy in a child's perceptions, an openness that attends to what is here right now. Many times the child is so involved with what has grabbed his attention, and an adult can upset that focus. The child's ability to attend is most often where the power struggles transpire because we are not only being logical, we are demanding a quick response. And that combination within adults puts the accent on getting done, performing, rather than the process-ridden focus of children. The power struggle is ultimately in the approach itself: adults want to see something done, while children want to investigate what makes it important and why would one thing be more important than my thing that is so great for me right now.

The challenge is in seeing behind the power struggle that we adults provide and into the meaningfulness of the child's determined choices. If we can expose for ourselves the as-yet unnarrated emotional truth behind the child's response, we are in a guidance moment that will make a difference in the child's understanding of self and other. With this effort the child need not resort to splitting out the difference between your power-truth and her felt truth. If that split does occur and is reinforced, the child builds a primary handicap that can insist that her center is likely faulty, and the new truth lies in who won the power. We are currently amuck in a society that is dominated by a power differential whose breeding and brooding began as young children, and whose loss of one's self trust occurred in the vulnerable connections with those we relied on.

Who might we be if we never have to lose our own emotional truths? We might be more likely to take in the beauty that is anywhere we walk and ask those questions that burst out of our minds. We certainly would enjoy curiosity in its creative allowances. Solution-thinking would have the stretch in it that provides thinking outside the box that we hope someone will provide when we are less able to bring it ourselves. Holistic health depends on trusting our own emotional truths while pondering the facts and truths from others.

CHAPTER 7

Andy: Being Found

In infant trauma, the baby has not been discovered. Dreaming has stopped; the baby no longer has the willpower to find or be found. I am called to see a child who is hardly 3 years old named Andy. This child stands apart whenever there is noise, a stranger, and any other "too-much" from the world. Andy has already received a diagnosis of Global Developmental Delay, particular to mental functioning. In addition, he has been identified as being on the autistic spectrum. His history: he was primarily alone for many months while his young parents partied downstairs. At 13 months he was taken into state custody. For a period of time he was placed in several foster homes. At around 2 years old he was put into a foster-to-adopt home with one of his siblings. At age 4 he was adopted into a household that understood the adoption process and the fragile child they were committing to. Later on, his youngest sister would join the family.

Compromised Trust

Andy has made do with very sporadic safety. His trust is compromised. He must meet new situations, of which he has far too many, with complete retreat. What a conflict this must present to the spirit: both a more urgent need to be found and a refusal to signal wanting to find and be found. Andy shows me immediately what he must do and be in order to "hold on," to stand still while the danger presents itself. There is no taking away his survival instincts of the situation. Andy is absolutely right about me: I am not safe. I've proven nothing in our introduction except that I might be another adult person that moves him about with no explanation. I might forfeit another hope that this home was worth his effort that "looking around" took. We are going to traverse the work of Andy and identify his developmental processes.

When I meet Andy, he stands near the door, looking for all intents autistic. It appears that he will not move, nor does he seem to register me. He takes up a frozen body posture and gaze, and remains in this position for around 20 minutes. I cannot imagine how unsafe I must be to him. So I begin to narrate this child's point of view in a quiet voice, saying something about where he might glance. I watch for signs that I am on the right track. This kind of narration is one of empathy and of tracking the child for any signals that might come from having opened up his senses. This tracking is not in the realm of success or failure. It is the mothering effort to be findable, to establish safety rather than results.

My aim is to show Andy that, without touching him physically, I perceive his whereabouts and what might be pulling on his frightened self. That first session lasts about a half hour. When Andy looks purposefully toward the door, I say he must need to see his mom, and we can do that together. He immediately moves toward the door.

Andy's neuropaths are hyper-firing and the message is Not-safe! Not safe! That message is all he can attend to, and so he appears to be autistic. His attention is so focused on safety that nothing else will wire or fire.

Knowing about a child's beginnings first comes to us in the intake, prior to seeing the child. The intake is vital, and yet it is only a handshake. The paperwork gives us an outline similar to landscape drawings, prior to ordering the bushes and trees that will take root in the soil. Most of the time we can return to our own experiences of having witnessed young children before, of having tracked each child through the debris while learning more and more about the interior tools of tracking. Each child has given us his or her own detailed knowledge of this landscape. At the same time, this is a new human being and we will establish a new set of tracks. We do not yet know where the trails will lead. We have our internal "maps," and the willingness to explore very troubled terrain.

It takes two sessions to feel safe enough together that Andy can begin to unfreeze, to regard me as potentially present. A little bit reliable, but not yet safe. That would take a long time of approaching one another, over and over. Here is where we begin again. I am pondering out loud, broadcasting for both of us what I observe, what might become a curious thing in the room, what is intriguing to me as I wonder out loud about Andy's meager movements. I increase my own sensate alertness to wonder about the room itself: Am I close enough? Too far? Does this matter? And this has to be done with a gradualness that is conscientiously slow. My intent is to develop a sense of emotional person relating to emotional person. But this is in the environment of a young child who has stopped trusting the motivations of adults and their meanings. And so my efforts are just that, efforts, and I have little response to let me know that I am correct.

Andy showed "lack of responsiveness to other people." He had a profound "lack of spontaneity and emotional reciprocity." Certainly he exhibited "extreme resistance or overreaction to minor changes in routines or environment." These symptoms come directly from the diagnoses for *Autism/Pervasive Developmental Disorder*. Let's hold these symptoms lightly while we walk about as near to Andy's interior map as we can be.

Those diagnostic definitions did little to give me the context of his neglect. In Andy's interior world of implicit memory, however, they were significant. They were like the breadcrumbs or more likely, the stones on the path that marked his baby encounters. Perhaps I appeared to be another holding place, like another foster home, that no amount of words would console. If that was the case, he would again lose the tenuous tether he might feel for this mother outside the therapy door. Or maybe I seemed to be the threat of a foster home parent who had begun to understand his "language of silence," a silence which was punctuated by wailing screeches when sudden noises occurred. I had done nothing to deserve the risk of trust that had fragmented during his pre-two experiences of chaos. I puzzled with these hypotheses as Andy and I started out on his path.

Instinctual Interactions between Mother and Baby

It is very hard to explore Andy's experiences in language since they did not take place in the language centers of the brain. It is about mutual recognition, an experience rather than an exchange. It is the act of what some philosophers call "worlding," which is the incubator of self-other recognition. That incubation occurs in the heart of a healthy caring adult.

Jessica Benjamin (2018) uses Winnicott to depict some of this foundational interaction. She describes recognition between mother and infant as "a constant element through all phases and events." She goes on to describe the requirement of both human beings engaged in this process of recognizing and being recognized. There is no single dance-step here: two are sending and receiving in this shared worlding. The mother is attuned, "devoted," Benjamin states, to the baby's own reach toward separation and the beginnings of self. She states that "reality is discovered, from the inside out, through being carried in someone's mind." The baby is unconditionally connected to the mother's devotion, while at the same time, sort of in charge of withdrawal times, excitement times, quieting periods. It's the mother's resonance and attunement that creates this mutual field. If we were to narrate the baby's experience, we would say that the mother obeys the baby. The mother is really tracking the baby's needs, following the baby's arousal/calm cycles that keep the baby's core within the government of the mother's own nervous system.

Benjamin lays out for us what is absolutely required for an infant to "hatch" into the world, this world that carries an individual forward into her own life. It is essential that this relationship is the baby's own, a given in the first months of life. She is not yet able to filter any of the feelings and body states that come to her and from her. Without this filter, this mutual unfolding and resonance, the baby must retreat. "Transformation of mutual fields" is the activity and the wiring up of self to self. It is only from this mutuality that a "me" will begin to build its own shape, with a body and feelings of its own (Benjamin, 1988).

This is also the task in therapy: to create and develop the field of mutual recognition. To do this, the therapist often has to start in a place without language and without the field of psychological time, which is the natural state of the infant. Prior to recognition is a sense of being not-present, then being *as if* under the child's control, and then the mutual dreaming. When infant neglect has occurred, we return to these earliest developmental requirements of the child. It will be up to us to comprehend what has not occurred in order to bring the potential of that developmental time, with all its complexities, into the therapeutic relationship.

Healing From the Interior

As the external world stabilizes through the consistent presence of another, healing begins in the interior with understanding the existence of past, undifferentiated feeling states. Understanding is not quite the right word because we might assume that this means that thoughts are present. The child is not thinking. She is tuning in and finding out that she is in contact through this attunement. Someone else is sending signals that say, "I'm still here. I can still find you. You are full of emotion. I am standing by and watching over your fullness." Play therapy explores stored feeling states that move within shared, felt wiring while building in a new template based on the potency and empowerment within the therapeutic relationship. This works as a back-and-forth modulating interaction: sustaining neutrality during high arousal (anxiety) and expressing the old feeling states during calmer interactive play (while relationship is available to soothe). The empathic-enough presence of the therapist contains past frightening and often shaming negative affects, which have come from the fused space of a parent and the parent's feeling states. The therapist's responsiveness will allow the child's nervous system to integrate new feelings. Dissociation moves to re-association, and the forces of anxiety, which have been fused with core life forces, gradually begin to pull apart and lessen, creating some access to the trust that had been compromised. Defenses relax over time, and the child begins anew, now learning to thrive in that same attunement which had proven so dangerous in the past. The child is now able to enter psychological time. What we are doing in therapy is re-uniting a "me" and a "you" into a safe "us" from which the child can find a self that is authentic and loveable. Development begins to move forward again. Love itself begins to merge with profound anxiety. This takes time and patience on the part of both the therapist and the child.

By age 1, Andy had experienced the failures and losses of loving that some of us have not known. He was born addicted to cocaine. Being born addicted causes an infant to be too numbed to hunt for and find the source of his survival, and to build on that source as the mother soothes him and guides him in attaching. The addicted infant's first experiences are not gentle, as addiction amplifies all senses. So the body that housed Andy, a very new body, began with sensory overload. Even holding these babies can be too much for their skin and the physiological and emotional antennae that the skin holds.

Trauma From the Lack of Mirroring

Infants who are born addicted, as well as those in addicted environments, typically lack the mirroring other. At some point in this un-relating where the hunting for the other is so compromised, dread settles in. Andy had been in a primarily disregarding environment for 13 months before he was put in foster care. His experiences had not been held together by someone who would hold experiences, render them tolerable, and provide him safety in his own interior experience. This is the first, foundational, requirement of the human being: to rely utterly on someone else to bring in the world in tolerable amounts of digestion and integration, over a period of months. Missing this filter, the self of the infant is vulnerable to fragmentation. Certainly, Andy had used some internal capacity of resilience to wait out a potential link to a potential adult. His safe experiences were sporadic and uneven. And Andy was very vulnerable to becoming stuck in his autistic protection since that armor could eventually become the overriding pattern of protective resistance toward others.

The more an infant feels the absence of the trusting other, the more he moves to extreme ends of response: either to do nothing and expect no one, or to fuss and cry out endlessly in an effort to be found. These increasing hyper-sensitive responses may seem to be the baby's own temperament, and that is often a part of the response. In neglect, however, the baby's reactions amplify the frustration coming from the parent, often leading to increased punishment and unavailability. Kalsched addresses this growing neurological chaos as "unbearable" in the infant. There comes to be a "breakdown," he states, in those processes "through which the child's volcanic affects might be humanized, metabolized by those caring for him." (Kalsched, 2013)

Andy's neurology will likely suffer from complete survival control: a reactive response that comes from the more primitive brain. Some might ask why I did not offer something, some interruption of his survival neurology, that might offer him my safety. Until I would be understood as safe, my "interruptions" were not likely to build the required connection between us. When frozen, Andy was unavailable to connection. His connection was to his own survival. My availability was to remain open and in attention.

When I first see him at age 3, I have been told Andy could stand more than an hour in one position in silence. His foster mother had worried that therapy might be useless, that Andy would continue to use this freeze pattern, well-known in trauma victims. Andy freezes in this way as a vulnerable animal might freeze when there is the scent of a predator. I need to understand myself in this hunter/prey relationship. His mother's seat outside the room is a constant throughout our work, and Andy periodically checks for her.

Andy's finger might twitch, or his eye might move a bit. I follow those movements, watching to see what his body cues me to. Perhaps these are the small signs that a mother guards as precious and responds to without thinking thoughts. I narrated what might be in the view of a movement, perhaps a doll or a noise in the street. I quietly add simple feeling words to what he might be peeking out toward, like moving over to the doll in question and wondering out loud if the "baby" is hungry, or wondering if that loud noise is a big truck or a little truck. My job, such as it is, is both to "be still" and to be Andy's movement. I continuously risk entering a silent zone, making myself potentially safe. Sometimes during a 50-minute period, Andy would follow the tone of my voice and begin to play. His language is soft and impossible to understand, and we guess at one another together. He does not look at me, and I feel like Medusa, whose presence could be suffered only through a mirror. What I internally feel is that I am flat like a mirror, with no 3-D characteristics. Being a sort of hologram, I am not involved in his play. I am being pushed about without being touched.

Andy had failure to thrive. Kalsched (2013), among others, has addressed how young children develop a self-care system to avoid dependency needs. Eating disorders can happen when bodily experiences have not been detected or understood. It may be easier to get our minds around the abuse itself, when it has been reported, than it is to comprehend that, for the child, intrusion occurs at every level of experience. While the mind works to closet off abuse, the body also escorts the child's self away from its pain and confusion. The confiscation of one's own authentic experiences maintains some darkened covering over the chaos of a polarity of thought: "I'm being hurt. But he loves me, so this must mean love." The hurt will be the aspect that is darkened. Andy hoarded food. If a dish of snacks was left out for family members to choose from when they were hungry, he would gorge on whatever he could hold. He also hid food everywhere. He pocketed small items in whatever handy spaces he had. His own understanding was that he needed to care for himself, thus maintaining his original experiences as current and unconsciously authentic. Food, from this vantage point, retained its survival requirement rather than being a resource that someone who was trustworthy provided the child.

Neglect in Me/Not-Me and Failure to Thrive

What has happened in so many of our wounded children is neglect of the developmental process of the me/not-me self.

In its place is a pre-mature non-dependence, a separation from others. Frances Tustin, in her work with autistic children, states that "such children do not transform sensations into precepts and concepts, and the basis for cognitive and emotional development is not established, or is established very insecurely. They have not developed 'psychic envelopes'" (Tustin, 2003). That second skin from the parent's emotional, interactive safety is such an envelope: the care of the other while the young child builds a sense of self. The child becomes a "me" through trustingly sorting out what is the "not-me" of the secure parent.

In neglect, the not-me has not been caring enough. There is no allowance for the infant to be dreamt into being. This means that the mother has been unable to mediate and delineate internal from external experience through attunement to the baby's needs. In a healthy relationship, the baby would emerge out of a shared space, simultaneously a dream-like and very real space, which is solidly held in place by the mother. The infant organizes his experience in this reliable transitional space, formulating a "me." But what I found in Andy was a faulty defense, an ability to be still and distant and unfindable. He had not yet experienced enough safety for a long enough period of time, to risk being together in a relationship while practicing being himself.

In having not been held in someone's mind, he was not available to his own mind. Andy's primary or authentic self was in there. That authentic person is the one who the mother mediates into being in the first year of life. It unfolds in relationship: in touch, in tones and smells, through the baby's body awareness of you-in-a-body. This learning about being in a body will be the hatching place when the infant is ready to absorb the not-me of the mother, therefore discovering the me of my own body. Slowly and surely the platform for a life is built in this relationship.

After a few more sessions of sporadic speaking towards me, Andy stops speaking again. For 6 weeks I show him that I have

Andy: Being Found

the courage to track his journey back into that nonverbal and unthought time in his life. I often feel as though I am all alone, speaking into a too-quiet space that houses echoes. It takes minutes in each week to warm up a frozen gaze, and then Andy might ritually take mother and baby miniature pairs and place them apart in the tray. His warming up face softens from that frozen gaze, and he seems to become more aware of me. I know he is covertly checking me as I quietly check in myself, showing soft emotions for his toy choices. His face has some muscle movement, as if he might speak but does not. I narrate that the babies would not and could not be by their mamas, that safety is being over here and over here. I narrate when mamas get closer to their babies and when they run away. And I narrate when the little mama sits and eats all the food, while the very big baby watches. Sometimes the very big little girl eats all the food while the little mama falls over in her chair. What is constant is that there exists no shared "digestion" of food or feelings. I am afraid I am giving in to trauma replay. The repetition of food and the mama's inability to be a participant in the play repeats, over and over. While I am concerned, I have learned from the work of other children that Andy's efforts regarding food, a mama and a gorging child will need to be safely seen by someone before that theme allows much movement or change.

As we travel through this terrain, Andy grows in his willingness to check up on me. He might put a mama over on a shelf or in a chair, while the young child sits at the table and eats both the child's and the mom's plates of food. As he creates this kind of constant scene, he looks at me as if to ask if I am getting what he is saying. Even though my paltry narrations seem like stabs in the dark, he returns to his work after I have punctuated that stillness with my efforts.

A ritual that Andy silently initiates during this time is that I draw him in detail. Not speaking, he brings a piece of paper and some pens to me and points to himself. I narrate that he wants me to draw him. He points at the colors we wear that are identical. I narrate that. He nods yes. Perhaps I need to draw him as the stand-in ritual for counting ten fingers and toes. At first, I try to engage Andy in drawing, but he makes it quite clear that this ritual is not his job, but rather, it is mine. He turns his back to my effort. I have already learned that this is akin to putting his hand up to silence me. There is to be no engagement until I am finished with my task, at which point he appears to be satisfied. It is my assignment in the hard work of repair. Perhaps my drawings of him at the table are the images of hope.

At times I feel a little bored and want to be in the more exciting place of witnessing play unfold. But later on, I understand that for Andy even to trust the experience of excitement internally, I need to be a little distracted, a little removed from the possibility of too much excitement that might occur with our growing attunement. Andy keeps this "me" busy enough so that "we" aren't too much for "him." This is what young infants know in their bodies, when they turn away momentarily from the mother's face, resting as it were. And then they return again to the eye-to-eye gaze of attunement. Neurology takes in these moments of devotion between baby and mother and earmarks them in the creation of trust and safety. Andy needs to approach this attunement on his terms.

And then Andy tries again. He will try at being safe enough to risk depending on me for a need. Perhaps I had passed the test of creating the newborn's attunement just a little bit. When he speaks again, it is to lay down pretend dollar bills and to point at the snacks. I narrate that to be fed, we need to buy food. I would accept his money and bring him some food. I give him dried apples. He spends a full 11 minutes chewing on dried apples, crunching away and staring at my face. I feel as though I am a sponge absorbing water and slowly taking on some kind of shape. Until then, I had not realized just how flat I had been. I feel and hear the fragileness between us, and wonder whether I (and he and us) would survive this. This crunching and staring into me happens in several sessions, each time taking 10 to 15 minutes of time, which is an eternity. After this, he begins sessions with staring at the shelf with snacks on it. I narrate his need; he waits for the agreed upon shared space. He needs a box of raisins for a pocket and a cereal bar to take to his younger brother. With enough fuel in hand, we truly start playing. Andy begins narrating his own story, which is gathered out of the threads of narration I had given over those 6 weeks. It becomes apparent that Andy has been listening all along. The word safety is our common word. He talks about the safe baby kitties most of all and uses a pink child as the mama.

There are many images and play scenes in the sand during this time. Nearly all of them address safety. For some period of time, Andy works away with two houses. At first, these two images in the tray are chaotic. Andy cannot seem to keep the miniatures standing up. All sorts of beasts come into the tray as soon as the houses appear. But gradually, without much narration from me, Andy begins to choose. Some of the dragons and lions come in and then exit again, with Andy shaking his head as if to tell himself they should not be so close to a house. He starts bringing in people to place around the tray. At one point he becomes organized enough to place an oddly mixed family around what he calls the "safe house," and then a fence around "the other house." After this, he is able to tell me that ghosts live in the house inside the fence, and families should not go in. We reinforce the boundaries around that house together.

Andy also goes through a period during which the houses are threatened from the outside. A fire engulfs the tray as Andy puts all the fire images from the room into the tray. In one of my many almost-failures, I pull in some firemen. Andy soundly refuses their use, saying that no, the fire must burn. In this effort, he does move the safe house into the wet tray, away from the heat. This little home becomes a new focus, and the not-safe house rarely enters after this explosive heat. Andy has sustained a very consistent metaphor, with its set of images: the lack of safety and the timing when he might entertain some safety. He is currently using all sensations of safeness to stay connected with me in order to believe that I might understand his powerful metaphor of safety/unsafety. Being seen through the metaphoric images played out in the sand, a child must keep going in the unfolding of his story until he experiences that someone has felt the metaphor. Then the child moves forward to next moments and meanings within a story that has already happened.

As Andy turns 4, his full intelligence emerges. Prior to this time, it may be that only Andy and I witnessed the growing order from his resilience. This is a child who had been given the diagnosis of mental retardation at 20 months. No one had quite known what he could comprehend. He understands months of the year, concepts of physical time, how to spell and write his full name. Andy and I both wear glasses. He comments on the shared realities in our lives, and then adds, "I love your glasses," or "I love your earrings." I mirror back our samenesses and our differences. He also begins using me as an aid in climbing onto stools to get what he wants from the shelves, a task he simply ignored when offered early on. As he becomes aware of potentially "using" my presence, he also resists that support, during which times, like a much younger child, he might become tipsy and lose his balance. His body is rather new at carrying a presence and a more creative focus to details around him. It is as if his body is narrating, "Hold on to me" while his hurts are saying, "Don't touch me yet." I do not think that early on he had really noticed me nearby, since this noticing was too painful for him. We are now taking small steps for short periods of time in the pre-one world of "usness." This world is, in my mind, a dream world, the *place in which a child builds an inner world through play and imagination. It is this space that shapes the creative self.*

The Sameness of "Us"

An important developmental process that Andy used was attaching himself to the samenesses of us. In this effort Andy had gone back to much earlier developmental phases and together we survived that reach of trust. In Andy's demand that I draw him every week, down to small details of the colors of his shoelaces, he established a memory bank. I felt at times that just in case I forgot something, there would be an image to remind me. He made sure I had the routine that helped me to remember. His "just-in-case" world housed many rituals that I needed to perform, to re-fire and branch from last week's trust into this week. Sometimes it felt as though what he dictated while I drew were really symbols of arms reaching out, across vast vacant areas, into this week, this moment, and the insistence that I remember.

Andy also took to bringing a stool to the window, where we played games while watching cars and trucks. From initially covering his ears with a look of terror, he could physically lean into me, taking advantage of my quiet neuro-body, while we agreed that that very loud racket was a very big truck, and very big things just had to make noise. The sirens were given shapes of ambulances and police cars, and those things eventually had a kind of concrete reason for making the noise they did. Andy would repeat the explanations I gave both of us: for instance, an ambulance meant that someone needed to hurry to the hospital to get better. I was reminded of the way in which infants at around 8 or 9 months, as they discover a world that their own motions might navigate, will constantly look back as they move forward, wondering how far the distance is between being at-one and being untied, as if an interior voice is saying, "I can move toward something new, but you can't go anywhere." We spent time re-wiring his hyper-sensitive antennae; or perhaps we spent time building insulation around nerves that had remained exposed and raw for the lack of parental mediation. At any rate, we were learning how to share a mutual space, an envelope that Andy could find somewhat reliable.

In a revealing scene, Andy takes the little safe house and again places it in the wet tray. He then uses his finger to draw a path looping about and ending on the far side of the tray. I have a clear feeling that Andy is not thinking about what he is creating, but rather, he is deeply playing. He stands back to look at it. Then he takes a little boy who is eating an ice cream cone and puts him at the place where the path ends. "He's just walking," he tells me.

In my mind, I note that there is no path back to the house, which bothers me. I wait a bit. We both look at the scene together. I ask, "I wonder where he is walking to?"

Andy looks closely. "He is walking to home." But Andy makes no further demarcation of the path heading back in the tray.

I say, "So he knows where that home is, and he can walk toward it, huh."

"Yes," Andy says. The image has spoken.

In that Andy was doing profound risk-taking. He had to choose, at some pre-conscious level, to come forward, approaching me with enough trust that I would remain while he reached out. Perhaps our more innate need while young, to depend on someone or something, assisted us both. Dependency is a dynamic that we can overlook in our need to run for healing. To heal an early wound that resulted from dependency not met, we must depend on someone being present while we remember and while we become somehow mindful of that failure. It is as if we must again fall into the void that was, feeling what it was like to not be held by someone before we can begin again. Winnicott calls this the breakdown that has already happened (Winnicott, 1971).

Andy could begin to imagine a map that sent him back home. But he did not yet have the stamina to carry out the feeling of the imaginable. Imagination is a direct consequence of attuned engagement of mothering: the infant gives out from within what cannot be digested. The mother absorbs this, and her digestion of its meanings are now palatable. She returns it to the infant in digestible form, in wholehearted form. This whole heart offers the necessary digestibility. Being whole is one of the definitions of embodiment.

By age 6 Andy is preparing for a break from therapy. He had been adopted during this time, and his forever mama had been receiving support through our Securing Connections Program. At home, Andy's food hoarding has greatly lessened. His anxiety still erupts when the old despair is present. But he accepts more of his mom's soothing and encouragement during his rough moments. He has internalized some personal calm when loud noises threaten his sensory alarms. Like any individual with a broken heart, there are vulnerable places. Andy seems able to acknowledge this.

Andy's eating disorder had mostly disappeared. Food still held intense responses at times, as it is a survival need in all of us. And when his survival past lit up neurologically, Andy needed to know he could control some of that urgent need. His adopting mom understood the existence of this and was consistently available when Andy showed signs of anxiety overthrowing him. At times, too, sudden loud noises still set off Andy's sensate sensitivities. It took courage to remain available to being found, even when an accident of internal alarm hit his neurology, and he howled sensing its potential danger. What was vital was to assist Andy in remaining present when that autistic withdrawal loomed when danger seemed too close.

What is important to think about here is not so much a "happy ending," but that the truth of the child's experience has found its beginning. Getting to that place and building what is useful has taken a tremendous amount of courage. The child has had to overcome patterns of false safety and weakened connections from having been with unsafe and unpredictable adults. This courage re-establishes dependency and trustworthiness. A child's trust has its own healing within it. We who spend time with children must comprehend what we are aiming for when this child in front of us had lost that faith in caring adults and how this child is letting us know where to look.

CHAPTER 8

Andrea: Development Within the Therapy Setting

I see a little girl who had flunked kindergarten because no one knew her capacity. Andrea will not respond to assessments that are given to her. She does not join in class discussions at all. She does not show that she is learning to read. She reveals no interest in daily classroom activities. There is no way to evaluate what she has learned at the end of her first year. Andrea is referred to therapy because no one knows what is going on. She does not play with friends on the playground; instead she spends time in a corner speaking with imaginary friends. In therapy, Andrea often sings her narrations to interactions between miniatures. She is a poet in her creations. As I take her creations seriously, she reveals those same entities she had spent so much time with, at cost to her academic and social growth. The friends and their environments take on stories that bring me quietly into a home life that no one would verify, but that seems filled with silent neglect. These friends gradually evolve into meaner entities, including witches and creatures with the power to zap her pretend friends into helpless servants.

It is useful to think of play therapy as having its own developmental process. The first stage, of finding one another in the playroom, is focused on building trust. We have already done an intake with the child's parents and have learned what they have defined as problematic or worrisome. While holding parent narrations as valid, we have not yet introduced ourselves to the child and the child's own perceptions. Remaining open to those meanings that the child has built is truly the first phase of therapy. As we are able to bring the child's own voice into the room and into relationship with us, we will have gained entrance to the deeper, crucial work ahead.

Early-Stage Treatment and Building Rapport

Setting the stage in which to collaborate in play is crucial. In some future playtime, words will become the bridge of differentiation between what is internal to me and what belongs to you, what is real and what is imagination, and what can be understood as two people mirror action together. For now, finding safety and trust is central. The therapist is the instrument, if you will, who carries the resonance in the room.

We can liken the therapeutic development of the child's work to the process of putting on a play. Feelings are put into the appearance of characters, rather than into words. Before a play can happen, there must be a narrative and a potential set of characters. In this way, the therapist enters the child's world from the child's point of view, learning from the stage director what the many nuances in the play are. What is not being said is also in the narration: the focus on the tray, the landscapes getting chaotic, toys being knocked over on the shelf. The child's unspoken actions provided enough details that the therapist might risk one sentence to help organize her story. "These lions are a family. The daddy lion has food. I don't know if he wants to share his food…" might be the first lines in the play. The child may look at you a bit, may add or correct what she has placed in the tray as an entry narration. This allows the child to know there is a construction beginning, and that she is in charge of its creation.

Andrea: Development Within the Therapy Setting

The therapist has offered the connecting link that she is available in the same way that a mother is available when the toddler points to a pasture and she names the animals he sees. Sometimes this may be as far as a child can go in therapy. Arietta Slade assures us that sometimes getting as far as understanding that "order *can* be created" is vital (Slade, 1994).

Early in treatment there is little, if any, challenge to what the child brings in as play themes. When the child resists options or reflective statements from the therapist, it is likely that the child does not yet feel the therapist's alignment. Interpretations, such as "That man is so angry. Daddies can really get mad" are not used. It is wise to trim down questions, as they can be interpretations in disguise. The therapist may not be aware of the disguise, but the child is clear about being asked what he or she is doing. Questions can enter the play sounding like "What would happen if that wild animal gets out of the pen?" The child knows full well what will happen and the danger he is facing. A child can often hear a question as "Would it be easier—better, more sane–if you went in the direction of my question?" Reflection and, later in the treatment, reframing are primary methods of communicating to the child what is going on.

Look for themes. When reviewing the child's process, the therapist will link up images used in play and track them across sessions. Track them as if there is a hidden pathway through the forest. Look for signals, threads, the child's glance at you when you did not expect it, movement toward and away from you, fallen toys. I had a little 4-year-old whose home life did not become safe during the time I was seeing him. I learned more from the toys he kept in his hand or dropped on the floor than I learned from what disorder entered the tray. The tray held his chaos while his hands and the floor held his efforts to organize himself.

As a child attributes to the toy babies, the witches, and the shouting his own perceptions and feelings, imagine the real-life situations reflected in the stories. Therapeutic ruminations are simply hypotheses that adjust as more understanding occurs about this child in this session. Importantly, listen for this particular child's unique and subjective way of processing and coping with those situations. Here, it is not merely particular events, but very significantly, the child's images and meanings tied to those events. The therapist remains open to changing her hypothesis by staying attuned to the personal metaphors and the shifts within the child's stories. Be cautious in heading prematurely to books for answers that might help in understanding the child's pathways. There is a kind of holding lightly to the pieces of threads we discover. If we erase our anxiety too fast and too much with another's insights, our own brains apply that salvation and we have succeeded in understanding someone else's ideas of the messages meant for us. We have not stretched our own tracking muscles. Over time, if we forfeit the possibilities that come from our deeper intuitive selves, the healing elements of our own inner tracker will be less present. The same goes for the play. While it is vital that we know the child's environments, do not hastily identify the child's selections in play as mere details of their outer lives. For instance, those chairs in a row are the classroom, and that loud voice is the teacher. Not necessarily. The child's choices cannot be so simplistically reduced. When we do so, we have run for safety, leaving the child alone in her perceptions.

Second Phase of Treatment

We transition into the second phase of work as everyone and everything in the room becomes useable. This is hard to describe. The toys now seem to have lives of their own, with their own feelings. The relationship between therapist and child has an authenticity to it that ushers in a sense of responsibility and protection for the child and his work. This phase is the longest

Andrea: Development Within the Therapy Setting

in its timing, as time now depends on the child's use of therapy. The themes and stories in the room are infused with metaphors that express the child's own meanings. We might, for example, internally question the use of the witches in Andrea's work: Why did the innocence of fairies get zapped by this darkness? We see a theme that takes shape over the weeks of sandtray work. Maybe we are asked to be the fairies, or maybe the witches. We may be asked to be the voice of an animal or a child as when Zack told me to "holler," giving voice to the child in the sewer. We attend to the child's own intentions in her choices of toys. These toys are now the activated storyline of the child's own self. Our task is to track the messiness of a story shifting as it adds and deletes characters and needs. The child counts on our own memory and our respect of the work that is unfolding.

During this vital stage in development, it may be possible to differentiate feelings: the snake is hungry; the baby is scared; the mommy is mad that the baby ate all the food. The child's own feelings become narrated in the feeling states of these characters. During this time, while feelings are getting their names, the interior is building some organization. A child might ask what a given miniature is feeling. The partnership of therapist and child figure this out together, with the directorship belonging to the child's own possibilities. Overwhelming feeling states are being broken into and broken down into manageable parts. This is the same process that occurs when the mother of a baby absorbs the overwhelm and sends it back to the baby in digestible form.

While asking the child to name their own feelings may well cause withdrawal and a return to disorganization, remaining in the play construction is safe (Winter, 1999). Children will create the time to narrate themselves as the directors when they have successfully navigated the construction in the mirroring and attunement of the therapeutic relationship. Slade states, "When we play with a child, we let the child know that we are there to be told... Children first learn to represent internal experiences because these experiences are first made real by another's recognition of them" (Slade, 1994). Symbols, which words really are, emerge out of the play and the us-ness of the relationship. In a very real sense, we are secured to ourselves through the shared attunement of play, of becoming ourselves through the recognition of another human being walking that mile in our shoes.

Once these pieces are practiced, of building a stage, choosing some characters (the toys as feelings and the therapist as co-conspirator), and listening for what these characters want to say, then and only then might reflection emerge in the play and in the relationship. The play now can be examined together (Winter, 1999).

Containment of the Unconscious in Play

Play happens to the child, from within the child, independent of consciousness. We return to the arena of dreaming together. Bromberg chases down the gut of this, saying that "The process of self-growth ... is not brought about *through* the relationship between patient and analyst. To the contrary, the source of therapeutic action *is* the relationship" (Bromberg, 2011). As we submit to feelings that are in need of discovery and expression, we submit to that "us": that not-conscious stage which is neither therapist nor child. We have entered "a shared personal field" (Bromberg, 2011). The therapist observes the play between figures and attends to their emotional quality. Paying heed to the internal responses within the therapist's self is crucial while simultaneously attending to the child's own unconscious energy at work in the play. If we provide a safe enough vehicle to the child's own truths, we have entered the field of co-transference. Children's more detailed processes will later focus on this dynamic.

The relationship is the space in which the child transfers her own perceptions, while the therapist learns who she herself is within the child's meanings through the roles the child assigns to her. When Zack told me to be the child who was sewer-sitting, the child's experience entered me, the catalyst. The assignments the child gives to the therapist assist the therapist in the transference, bringing us the feelings behind the images. It is important to participate in the mutual field while not doing one's own work with the child. For instance, the therapist has a poor childhood/parent relationship. The therapist is told to be 5 years old. The therapist becomes very heatedly a 5-year-old, talking back because that insistence, that transference, is in the room. There will be no space for any growth in the child, as the two are merely replaying the shared child/therapist perceptions.

In a good-enough therapeutic encounter, on the other hand, the therapist experiences the 5-year-old sensation of anxiety and lack of voice. The therapy can now bring an exploration of this anxiety and loss of voice into the room, seriously playing out the interchanges that the child brings. In the hard work of play, the therapist emotionally attunes to the child's experiences, and brings regulation and an openness to change. The therapist in the above example presents both the child's five-year-old feelings and the child who would have experienced an authentic adult. The combination of relationship and the child's natural environment of play will offer the maximum opportunity of healing. Feeling the sensations the child has brought into relationship, the therapist is able to amplify and express these sensations, while remaining in touch with the child's own perceptions. What is present in the therapist, then, is the "me" *and* the "us" of this working unit.

During this time, Andrea continues in her sing-songing world of poetry. I am becoming involved with her trance states that keep her creativity safe and seemingly out of reach of something else. Looking back on this time in our sessions, she was opening up her hidden world to me while continuing to disallow any reality checks. Any narration on my part about the shadowy creatures entering the play makes the play itself come to a halt. Andrea's world is detached from human engagement. In that sense, she is no longer using imagination. This had become a swollen private world of fantasy.

When a child has experienced too little wiring-up as an infant, fantasy replaces relationship and attunement in the service of a kind of falsely soothing organization of self. As the child uses toys, and eventually discovers this safe relationship, fantasy is placed in the toys, which are themselves the props to the therapy relationship. Ignited by a growing trust, fantasy slowly becomes imagination, and in the arenas of safe relationship and imagination, the child turns back to authenticity. Imagination is relational, while fantasy as used in this context disconnects.

To allow others to attach means that she would experience a lack of safety. Perhaps she would be found, or found out, as not being safely tethered to a more interactive parent-child relationship. Where this danger comes from, and at what strength that danger occurs, is left out of reach. I choose a parallel plan: I bring in a journal just for Andrea, and with her permission, begin writing down her free-style poetry. If we are going to remain literally out of this world, I need to at least capture the filmy constructs that sing, light-footed, in the room. As we gather her together in this journal, she starts drawing pictures of her words in this journal, and true feelings enter.

At one point, she suddenly blurts out her own sense of disgust that her parents got so drunk the previous night that her mother had to crawl on the floor to take care of herself. Just as suddenly, Andrea clamps her hands over her mouth and begs me not to remember what had slipped out. "Forget that! I didn't say anything!" Andrea is panicking. Her gesture communicates to me how stern she had been in not saying anything about her home life, not risking saying her real thoughts because she had committed to this protection of her parents and her primary attachment figures.

Andrea: Development Within the Therapy Setting

As she lets go of this powerful editor in her, Andrea shows that she has mastered the goals of first grade, after all. She knows how to read and to solve some math problems. The defense she had built was taking enormous amounts of energy every day. Her imagination begins to remain in service to who she is, a very real, very creative child. She had used her own talents on behalf of a barrier rather than on behalf of its authentic presence: that of creativity.

In play therapy terms, let us say we are in the middle phase of treatment and have found common feeling in many of the child's choices of miniatures in play. Being in the receptive space, the child goes to Star Wars figures. The therapist waits openly and without questions while the child carefully selects Yoda and Darth Vadar. Both therapist and child are playing together with the current focus on these images. How the child settles these two figures will articulate many possibilities. Vadar might grow to be less and less the definitive dark lord from a movie. How those two images engage now in this session, whether they return and how often, whether in their future one slowly wins or whether they befriend each other–all this is the mind of the child hoping to be understood and the therapist wanting to know while not cognitively making assumptions. The effort here is to convey each child's use of objects as subjects, as dream images that correct, re-align, and make new meaning of old wounds. While the therapist is looking at toys, she is comprehending active images. We are thinking nouns and acting on verbs. The psyche of the child is not separate from their surrounding world and is closer to the act of dreaming than logic.

One of Andrea's final trays holds the tensions she had held internally. She makes a kind of bank of many flowers at one end of the tray. Into these big flowers, she nestles plastic eggs, the kind we use at Easter, that open up to hold goodies. Inside one of these she places babies. Then she brings one of the witches in, who is going to harm the babies. At this point in the therapy, Andrea has recovered her own voice that speaks through the characters in her story. She adopts the voice of the scary witch and resolves to play out the danger itself. I sense it is time to intervene. Andrea is still in an environment that has not resolved drug addiction, although there are now state helpers in the home, coaching the parents. I take one baby and become the protector. She struggles with me, saying the witch will not hurt the baby. I say that this baby has already experienced enough sadness and scariness, and I do not know if witches tell the truth.

Andrea's shoulders fall as she sighs, and she tells me to put the baby back in the shell. "She's got to be born, and I promise the witch will not be able to hurt her."

"Okay," I say. "But if I see any harm, the baby will come in my arms again." Andrea puts the baby back in the flowers, inside the egg. She creates a ritual of one of the miniatures who had represented one of her imaginary playground friends. This quiet figure taps at the shell. With some tension, Andrea opens the shell, pulls out the baby, and adjusts the flowers so that this baby is sheltered in a circle of growth. Andrea and I have somehow passed through a last requirement: that I stand firmly on the side of protection while this baby girl is "re-born" into a protective landscape.

Andrea steps back and observes her work. "This is beautiful, isn't it."

Impairments From Trauma

Trauma generally impairs the healthy integration of unnarrated emotions and sensations. Play therapy assures that these memories can be witnessed and then narrated. It is not the languaging but the organization of feelings into thoughts, thoughts into shared understanding, shared understanding into the grace of being in a relationship that trauma originally invaded. Relationship as therapeutic action has carried the child's hard work toward a new sense of self held within safety.

Andrea: Development Within the Therapy Setting

What potentially makes expressive sandtray and art therapy useful is the fact that the child uses the materials for inter-projective drama while using the relationship as a safe place in which to recreate early developmental phases. The toys are the medium; the relationship is the affect regulator. Really, the relationship is everything else: all that wiring, firing, and interconnection that ultimately secures attachment. The interior and exterior worlds are renegotiated together. Safety is always the first go-to, and calming that core requirement, safety, lies in the limbic system. In good-enough play therapy, the child returns to primal spaces, since it is the limbic regions of the brain that are firing the implicit meanings.

Daisy, 4 years old, is still in foster care, waiting for a placement. She suffers from acute failure to thrive. Food seems unable to pass through her throat before it comes back up.

Daisy's fierceness is to be reckoned with. She tells me I am two, and sits me down with a plate of sand. At this point, she begins yelling at me: "Eat it! Just eat! No talking! Be quiet!" I had not yet said anything. The emotional disorder is penetrating, and I feel unable to eat or to think about eating. From this "us" connection, I simply state, "I am a little afraid to eat. When you yell at me, I become afraid."

I am told again to be quiet. I say I am trying to listen to being quiet, but I am still scared. "Okay, okay. Just sit there then. Eat the food." Daisy's voice had calmed a little. She seems to be thinking about the idea of being scared. We have stepped a little closer to her own failure to thrive. I have been able to stay with the sensations she threw into the room, without triggers in myself around being yelled at, being forced to eat, or being helpless. In that set of circumstances, we are both successful this time. I have remained present. Daisy's implicit memories that told of indigestible experiences have entered the room. Her memory has not caused harm.

The heart of the child's implicit realities is communicated within and through the play metaphors the child has chosen. In the child's social environments the same metaphors can be occurring in behaviors. For instance, the child has a history of abuse and neglect. The metaphor selected early in treatment, which guides the therapist into the child's inner world and defenses, is the sick, in-bed, mom. In behaviors, that "sick mom" image is expressed in the child's school, in weak trust toward teachers and other school personnel. According to the child's expectations of trust, adults seem to be weak and unable to mirror this child. It is important that the therapist learn the congruency between environments in which the child travels. The therapist need not narrate the child's use of this difficult image to others outside the playroom. However, wondering if the child has experienced adults as not seeing her (and therefore feeling unuseable to the child) will assist in enlivening teachers and other school players to approach this child's neediness. In settings outside the playroom, the therapist represents the child's resistances toward adults that had been revealed through the work of the sick mom, and thus adult illnesses. A mom who is in bed is a parent who may not be present to the child's own needs. One potential question this child may be carrying is, "Are all adults sickly? Do they need my help like my mama does?" This child may show a lot of anxiety in her school when she needs something and she has no idea who to rely on and how to present her requests.

In understanding the meaning of the stories and metaphors that a child creates and uses, we need to recognize that the material will incorporate both the child's interior worldview and their psychosocial conflicts. These constructs are relevant to particular stages of development. Through them, we might get closer not only to what has happened, but also to how old this child was developmentally when it happened. Developmental ages are not the same as linear ages, since oftentimes we are spending time with children whose hurts occurred at pre-one states of development. We will go back, with the child directing us, to earlier unfinished growth.

Repair and Attunement

Daisy continues to drive the both of us through her deep fears of abandonment. In session, we return again and again to the "dining room table," to eat. Daisy examines with me the harm of being yelled at, and then being left to eat alone. She scans my face, seeming to remain uncertain that I get it. She also wants to know how to calm herself, and my own calm while these emotions visit builds a map for her. We go into the art room, where we begin a new theme of baking.

Daisy discovers that there is plethora of ingredients to mix together! A lovely mess. She takes delight in the brews she creates. At one point, she insists I try it, to see if it is edible. I purposely amplify that I pretend-try it. "Not too bad," I say. She laughs at my ambivalence. Together we find enthusiasm and play in this odd mixture and its likelihood for food. Daisy insists that we save it as is. I put the container with its greenish-gray mess into a cupboard.

The following week I pull it out for us to investigate. It seriously reeks. We both make an awful fuss over it. "What is it?" I exclaim. "It's throw-up!" she shouts. I heartily agree. Now Daisy wants to keep it, for sure. The following week it is moldy. Again, we identify it and enthuse on its transformations.

What is profound about this ongoing exchange is that Daisy starts eating real food more readily. Her hunger button in her brain has started up again. We had made her eating, the terror, and her vomiting, sacred. What is stuck now relocates in image, where its story is more tolerable. We could start again.

Daisy had shown an intense focus on food and the emotional atmosphere while eating. She brought her needy focus to a new examination when she threw together ingredients that eventually gave her throwing up an image. I hadn't prepared this play experience as a therapy goal or treatment plan. Daisy and I together created the movements she needed to befriend something that had deeply frightened her.

Maria Kendler, in an article for the *Journal of Sandplay Therapy*, summarized some important points to therapeutic play. She had been focusing on the problem of "What if nondirective therapy isn't helping?" and she goes into the essential ingredients in attunement repair. She addresses the primal chaos in a child who has not received infant care. She points out that it is up to the therapist to return to these beginning levels and to meet the child there. The position we take, for instance, in physical distance and closeness is so important to a child. The therapist will find the space in which some charge or current between the two continues, not too much and not too little. This exchange of physical/neurologic distance lets the therapist know what the child needs from his body memory. How we express our own attunement, and when, offers assurance to the child that the relationship is safe and is carrying her, the child, in its arms (Kendler, 2017).

As Daniel Stern states, the mother's facial expressions, as a reflecting mirror, organize the child's emotional experience. The young child uses the mother's face as a representation of his own feelings and can take this representation in until a much later time when he can name his own feeling states (Stern, 1995). We can accompany the child's play with matching sounds and facial expressions that reflect the emotional value of the play, providing a deep congruency when the child is playing with personal dynamics present in the tray.

The therapist is the memory and the moderator of the play. Through an active and responsive attunement, the therapist is charged with calming over-activity and bringing in the power of feeling when under-activity occurs. We can refer to this as building self-states that the child learns about, finds safe, and

Andrea: Development Within the Therapy Setting

absorbs the use of. It is like building a weblike construct from within the child's own self that connects and designs a wholeness that might reveal the face of the child's own uniqueness.

What is vital to understand is that, for a child, the safe therapy relationship and the toys as vehicles to interacting in relationship are not logically separated. When the child senses that she has been found, she says, "Come on then. Let's go to where I have not been understood. Let's see if I can *get* understood." The toys actually become feeling states that carry the relationship down into the narrow tunnels of implicit memory.

Our commitment as play therapists is to gain the stamina to carry and contain the unknown, to be able to play in the space between one another in a manner that reveals through trust who this other human is: the child in one's office. There is nothing more important than who this child is.

So, what does it take to be in relationship with these deeper edges of the self and other? What are the dynamics that let us know that we are in its territory, that we are "with it?" More often than not, this does not feel very secure, and it should not. It is more a feeling of vulnerability, of falling toward another human being. We first meet a person and they appear as our judgment states: old, young, wrong mustache, stern looking. Soon we find ourselves with a different set of eyes, which reflect curiosity about them: Why do they look up like that? What are they seeing? What makes her look so sad? If this has not happened within a couple of sessions, we may need to get out of our own way. We want to gather together a mutual field, a reflective place, before we can head out with the child into the child's world. We are actually falling a bit in love, you might say. Some amount of elixir must be present for us to be the right person for safely falling toward together.

This is the space to hope for in the healing of trauma. Winnicott tells us: "It is only when alone (that is to say, in the presence of someone) that the infant can discover his own personal life.

The pathological alternative is a false life built on reactions to external stimuli. When alone in the sense that I am using the term, and only when alone, the infant is able to do the equivalent of what in an adult would be called relaxing. The stage is set for a self-experience. In this setting the sensation or impulse will feel real and be truly a personal experience" (Winnicott, 1971). To comprehend the process of hatching from a shared reliable relationship, we repeat and update this mutual personal space again and again, holding the child's self in order that this human being has the power and safety to be certain of this individual self.

A shared understanding between therapist and child brings about an ability to be in the play and then step outside together long enough to enhance, amplify, think about what is going on. After much work together with a 5-year-old boy named Todd, who had been abandoned by both parents, Todd looked at me as he again pulled a miniature of a child who is crying from the shelf. He said, "You know, there are many me's inside me. Some of the me's know about her crying. Sometimes I know that my parents lost me, and I got hid by being Emily. Sometimes I am not Todd. I think people should know this, but they don't. How come?" His question was one of deep reflection, with many levels that would need yet more work to unfold. But the meanings had come together and had allowed me a large doorway into his feelings. We could begin slowly to reflect on his own wounds that made him question if being Todd would become ok.

When this capacity occurs, to step outside the play together, and then back in to add and enhance the play, we enter the final stage of therapy. There will be many rehearsals, frustrations, and practicing as the characters do not always remember their parts in the story's narration. As the child practices through many variations in the play, she reviews her own empowerment to remain identified as her authentic self. We can close the therapy with the child's understanding and recognition of being a separate self.

CHAPTER 9

Mona: The Wounds of Abandonment

Not long ago I had the grace to spend time with a baby about 2 months old. When he woke and found me, his not-mother, standing by, he was indignant! Angry, he cried out as if I was supposed to fix this mess we were in together. I circle back now *to aggress* and its essence. To aggress, as noted in chapter four, is to "start an attack," which then broke open to "a step, stage, degree." In Latin, the ad- prefix means "to, toward." This baby was clearly attacking this strangeness with all the might in his little body, where he *felt* my otherness. His aggressions, such as they were, were meant to resurrect his mother and find safety. As an outsider, I needed to convince him that I might do for a short period of time.

Aggression and Attachment

Aggression, from this point of view, is crucial. It is part of the fabric, the muscle and tendon, of attachment. Perhaps the baby's call for the absolute other, because that other is still a symbiotic *me*, is not heard in its fullness. Attention is not directed to this primal need. The baby initiates a premature separation. This is what happened with Andy, whose work we touched in on in chapter eight. He felt too little stretch in the fabric.

Andy comes to play therapy. I am to attend to Andy's silent hollering. To break into what play therapy really may offer, we might open up that dry noun: attend. *Attend* in its root means "to stretch," which approaches "direct one's attention to." To stretch moves to "extend… to stretch out before" and "to cause to endure; to hold on to; tender; a tendril or tendon…" This becomes rather useful and important to those of us who hunt for each child's truths. We are compelled to reach across spaces often unknown to our selves, tolerating our own misgivings in order to trust the child's desire to be found. We stretch out with tendrils of belief toward a child who wants understanding. We hope to hold on to, endure, and succeed.

I am called upon to *stretch*, to push out beyond my mental knowledge to find this singular child. In this effort, he is the unique infant that was in someone's arms, or not, yelling indignantly until the aggression was too much for him, and he quieted himself. My stretch will need to go to the place where Andy stopped stretching and stopped believing that he would be heard. Andy will take me to that place if I do not prematurely do what he did: create silence as a form of protection. As I remain open to Andy's markers along his path of repair, I know Andy will show me where his danger increased, where it left him abandoned, and what he did to survive those losses. Andy will eventually make use of the very same aggression he needed as a young baby to demand that I be present. With my attending, the two of us create the strong tendons and muscles required to bear up to holding a human being. And all of this is narrated without words. What are we listening for when we are not listening for words? This is at the heart of play therapy: this use of two selves who approach one another in a world strewn with so many dialogues.

Silence and Neglect: Selective Mutism

There were definitive places where Andy marked his baby losses within the ongoing map of his work. He had come to see me because of his early neglect. His environment had been terribly disorganized. His entry into the playroom spoke volumes to me about not expecting my attending, about giving up on finding dependability. Andy's first major breakthrough came when he that let me know how silent his infant world had been. Andy had chewed away at the dried apples while staring at me a good 10 to15 minutes. The cost of not being heard in his indignation had left a stunning silence, the baby Andy not knowing how to gaze into the mother's face nor to look away from the mother's face for rest from that intensity. Andy brought his frozen gaze into the room that day, while he stared at me with little acknowledgement. Shortly after that, he began arguing with me nonverbally. He would point to the food, and I would narrate his pointedness. He refused to let me know what he needed verbally and to speak was still too threatening. I had to *find out*, like the new mother who wonders if anything she is doing is right.

It may be, however, that in Andy's refusal to speak he was actually setting up a place for himself in trying to find out whether or not I was safe. In an odd sort of way, his temporary mutism enabled him to be in charge of his vulnerability. He found he was able to get help from me in accessing resources while at the same time he remained in his babyness of not using words. We can make hypotheses about this, while not losing track of Andy's meager choices. Maybe as he went to past developmental needs, he became congruent with the language that very young soul held. Or, maybe some form of aggressive/stubborn health showed up, signaling to me how much it would take to earn his trust.

After this, Andy brought miniature play food into the play, using the dollhouse as the setting. The food was huge and flooded the toy table. The tiny story mother sat by while the child ate it all. And as the child ate, the mother was removed and put several feet away, sitting on a shelf, disconnected and unable to witness this child's needs. The child connected to food when the mother disconnected. How slender that tendril was. Very little nourishment from the mothering space. The food was so large in its need, and the mother was so small in her presence. I remember my own anxiety when the mother was uselessly placed on a faraway shelf. I wanted to talk about it. But my impulse to talk really came from my urgency to decrease that pain of physical separateness. And yet, each time Andy repeated this distance between his play mother and child, he absorbed just a little more aggression, a little more willingness to emerge as himself. He was in charge of the distance to the mother as he painfully showed me how far she must sit. Three months or so in, Andy created the house-on-fire scene. This was done in silence, with no fire sirens and no one calling for help. The baby was on the second floor. Firemen could not endure the heat. Repair and salvaging were still too weak. The details of danger could be seen and represented, but too little muscle existed to exercise finding the baby. I recall that day with Andy: I wanted to convince him that the firemen knew how to do their job. Could he let them into the burning house? I was able to keep quiet, while inside I felt a heavy agitation. I wanted both of us to save that baby. Perhaps I held the urgency while Andy held the inability to save anyone as yet.

Later, Andy made use of two homes in the sand: one was safe and one was scary. Over time he built up the safe home, adding a fenced-in yard, some animals, other children. As I maintained my stretch, Andy could be seen, through his metaphors, risking some stretch toward me. The pathway he designed, in heading away from the safe house, stretched between us. He said it was "a map." The child would walk back on the map to the home. The child had found his own stretch, his motivation to look toward a safe home and to hope that he was also looked for from this home. Andy and I had updated his loneliness to a current reality of having people in his life, others who stretched to find him, who attended to him. Andy had bundled together a myriad of feelings that exposed themselves in this singular image: the child on the road home, eating. Although this was a positive image, the child did not move toward the house. But Andy could now *imagine* that he/the child *could* move.

What does all this say about being child therapists, and for that matter, therapists with people of any age? "We need relationship to each other to get to this power in us, to develop this capacity to make something of our experience and to accept that experience makes something of us. This capacity does not come into being unless it is recognized and responded to by an other, someone who looks at us with a gleam in their eye, seeing us, prizing us simply because we are, contemplating the good of us, our being. We are dependent on this other" (Ulanov 2007).

Dependency is contingent upon this gleam in the other's eye. *Contingent* here points us back toward dependence: "Liable to occur but not with certainty; possible." Perhaps, dependent upon the attention given and received, this relationship spins itself forward at deeper levels than we might dissect in discussions and diagnoses. Ulanov goes on to say that trauma enters our worlds when overwhelm occurs, "before we are able to make something of the experience or register that the experience makes something of us" (Ulanov, 2007). We therapists give full honor to each scrap as it surfaces in image, dream fragment, felt exchange, and we hold them together until each one becomes useful again.

"Don't Look at Me" and Neglect

I began working with Mona before she was 5years old. Mona had spent almost her first three years in an orphanage in China. Her attachment to her new parents was very ambivalent, and oftentimes disorganized. The parent intake revealed a child whose behaviors fought with parent efforts at feeling safe.

Her first interaction with me involved Mona creating a bed out of blankets in the therapy room, laying down silently on them, and then flatly telling me, "Don't look at me." Mona immediately and confrontively seemed to put us both into an alignment with her past. I felt useless. Mona had spent much infant time horizontally and in the concretely defined space of her crib. Now, from this position, her needs and her sense of emptiness came into the room and into our relationship. Mona began the first few sessions in this "remembering" position with a bottle, both acquainting herself to my presence as a potential relationship and as a way of remembering the scraps of herself: remembering what had been omitted for her survival. Her remembering was in her body, in a position of being forgotten. Her demeanor was one of obstinacy, and she could have been diagnosed with oppositional defiant disorder. Her energy, of being laid out there on a blanket staring at me while telling me to "not look," was very painful.

Once Mona begins to sense that I had seen her and had felt enough of the silence of her babyness, the rage of this early omission in her life makes its presence. Food had been an important inclusion, both in the beginning of her life and in the beginning of our relationship. Mona had made a ritual of my cutting up an apple, peeling it properly and to her critical eye, and then eating it slowly and carefully. In a session 2 months into our time, she taunts me with apple-slice sharing. Both major parts of the child are now present: the one wanting to be generous and to connect; and the other, angry, needy, unbearable. Mona attempts to spit on me when I calmly assert that she cannot eat parts of the plastic that had protected the apple.

Overwhelming Monsters: Implicit Memory

Mona's interior monsters were in the room. Both she and I needed to first figure out how to tolerate their presence, and then to work together on safety. Mona had "set me up" to confront her lack of safety in eating something that was not food, and that was instantly a safety boundary. In establishing this boundary, Mona now had something to fight with. It looked and felt like me. Meanwhile, I felt the effort in myself to correct her and to make this a power struggle of manners. I "took in" the engulfing sense of rage in Mona, that she could overthrow me and this seemingly incorrect relationship I continued to offer. Now we had something to "argue about!" which was not comfortable at all, for either of us. What is crucial here is that if I could not remain in "our" discomfort, surely Mona could develop no stamina to argue with her monsters. Both of us needed to be terribly uncomfortable, with Mona relying on me to know what to do about it. This is that absolutely vital developmental place of the baby's narcissistic rage, pushing him into "extremely high levels of arousal, which are beyond his own modulation" (Schore, 2003). If Mona was to sense those old terrors in the room, she must also sense my own capacity to stay attuned and to modulate for her while she found this muscle and figured out how to use it. There we were, an infant and a mothering person who needed, for the first time in Mona's life, to weather full-strength feelings.

I align myself with that part of her that desires care. Mona and I are very in touch with one another now, which is triggering Mona's fears that I will soon leave her alone. This is an implicit memory that is defended by her limbic system of fight-flight. This memory is here in this moment of my care. I hypothesize that she has moved into the fight/flight induced by her trauma. Mona has already shown me she is dysregulated. Sensing my alignment, Mona releases a deeper disconnected and disorganized memory. The monsters, Anger and Coldness, stomp about in the room. As I tell Mona I could not retrieve the plastic if it were to go down her throat, she begins racing around yelling, "I'm vomiting on you! Yuk!" while making snarling sounds. I can "see" the entity who both wants to and could not tolerate being seen. Still in the grip of Mona's early implicit experiences, I am fast becoming the infant who had had too little attending, too little recognition of being one special person. Mona's felt memories are here, right now. Because they are so full of terror, I am that baby, while Mona expresses the feelings that belong to that baby. By now Mona's face is distorted, full of rage. Her body seems not a part of her voice. A baby crying with a profound need to be held is present. I begin the unsteady process of carrying that rage of the traumatized infant who is forcing her way into the room and into me for containment. It is too soon to calm her, as she has worked so hard to let me see this rage.

With strong affect, I voice both the vomiter and the hope between us. "It stinks so bad. If you throw up on me, you really might not like me. If you like me, you might get hurt. And, I do like you. This vomit is all over me and it stinks badly and I am really sad."

The charged space between us also marked the earlier powerful space between mother and baby. The baby is all subject, while the mother is preoccupied with holding steady while the baby hunts toward the connections she offers. This overlapping implicit reality of the mother/therapist is re-accepted and given room to manifest (Cattanach, 1992). When a young child goes toward her losses and abandonment, the good-enough therapist stretches out to attend to the unfinished rage, the calling of a baby whose language had not been heard. When this occurs, we are not in psycho-drama, but rather, we *are* the experience. The child tries again. The effort of trying to locate trust makes room for the emotional guardians that had been a false safety.

It seems as if my endurance of "vomit" all over me moves us along in this hostile environment. Mona eyes me defiantly, wondering perhaps how I manage to stay so stinky with her aggression, fear, and emptiness. All of a sudden she states, "Here!

I'll get it off. (She scrapes at my clothing.) Oh! Now it's on BOTH of us! Disgusting! Gross!"

I stand up and move toward the bathroom, saying, "It is gross. All that goes in the toilet." She follows me in, we shake ourselves off, and she flushes the toilet.

While we stand near the toilet together, Mona tells me that China is very far away. I agree. She asks me if I would go there and get a baby. I say it is not too far away for me to get a baby. She asks if I even know where China is. "I do," I say. "It takes plane rides," she tells me. I agree. She accidently calls me Mama during this time, and I do not put any attention on this slip. Her experiment with that powerful word needs emotional acceptance from me.

So much tension remains after such an intolerable visit from the monsters and from the past. Following this level of discharge, a child must express some potential regulation in a medium that absorbs some of this articulated effect. Otherwise, reenacting and making literal that experience will likely happen in some form outside the therapy room. Near the end of this particular time, Mona painted. This material was soothing to her, and as I remained close by, we reestablished our caring-people beliefs. She was genuine and polite. The mutual field between us was marked with consideration, perhaps a close companion to recognition.

When a child has not succeeded in early developmental stages, a primal gap remains that she must attempt over and over with increasing rage. Oftentimes children who have not been recognized as individuals remain caught in this impossibility of other people being mere extensions of one's self. This is inauthentic power, and builds upon its own isolation, which can lead to personality disorders. The therapist must see that to enter into the child's inner world of fear and survival is to enter into hope. This is radical hope, that makes or breaks the longing to be found. Here is the deepest use of our compassion: to find out what it is that this child keeps repeating and to unmask the terror that keeps wanting us to find the child buried within that repetition, that requirement that the child be somehow understood. The hope lies in the child's continued effort to be found.

Metaphoric Expressions of Neglect

As the child senses that we are safe "enough," she approaches the realm of imagination, of "imaginal acts" (Schwartz-Salant, 1998). This approach is, for the child, the metaphoric language that carries her story toward us. We will not receive a direct story of her experience as an infant. Rather, the language of images in the tray will reveal her own understanding. Our focus moves away from knowing and toward the radical hope itself, the effort to understand. To enter this field, we must give up or loosen up ego control to a high degree, but not to the extent of fusing with another (Schwartz-Salant, 1998). Something more is needed, a desire to experience this mutual field in ways that may surely reveal the limitations of any logical concept one had of a particular interaction. Mona and her aggressive monsters had heard about hope. They were Mona's protectors against more harm. They had listened in to the two of us fussing about relationship and safety. They were determined to help me find Mona in her abandoned place. The vomit and Mona's effort to disgust me were her own feelings of not deserving care. If I could "stand in" for her raw feelings, there would be someone both sharing her experience and having the muscle to carry her toward the hope of a safe relationship.

What do we mean when we speak of this mutual or relational field? It is that charged location in which two people are working together. We can say it *is* the relationship, and yet it is a bit more or other than that. The relationship itself builds the field, and it is what occurs in that relationship that sustains this field. We might imagine the therapist as a tracker. In the wilderness, she finds the paw print, the first effort on the part of the child to be found. In the scree and dry rubble, there is little to assist in finding a series of prints. She listens; she waits. As her instincts access a different sight, she can see the brushed-aside leaves where this child/animal entered the thicket. She has now entered the animal's motion, but she is not yet a part of his travel. Then the tracker/therapist moves because she has the language of who this entity is. She has done some sort of internal intuitive and imaginative calculation. The therapist/tracker understands how this entity chooses the path he has taken. The decisions the child had made for protection remain unconscious and left deep in the folds of implicit memory. Can all this be talked about, be given a generalized road map? No.

After many more sessions, Mona could contain polar ends of being a person a bit more often: her old unloved self and her newer relational self. She continues to confront and rage toward me during a session and hug me at its end. She taunts me with gestures of peeing on my carpet and learns that I move into her taunts and can witness her old, wild self fighting with the new self. In one session she throws her panties at me, and I simply catch them, tell her to go to the bathroom, and name the underwear as belonging to her in a very practical way. She asks if they are for babies.

"No," I say. "They are good panties for 5-year-olds."

She becomes confused emotionally and again calls me mama. She asks me why kids come to this place.

"To share their feelings together with me."

"Like when their moms go away?"

"Yes."

"Like when a brother and mom and dad and sis go away?" More discussion. Then: "I am going to make a self house. Don't look at it. (Remember her first sessions of lying on a 'bed' and telling me not to look at her.) It can be pretty scary. These—scary *teeth—But don't look! Just think about it. Do you like scary teeth or not-scary teeth in this house?"* She continuously reminds me not to look, that this is too scary. Silently she cuts the teeth out, ragged edges that do look like shark teeth. She whispers the letters of her name as she writes them along the teeth sections of her self house.

In this place a powerful connection comes to life, and it is held in a strong container. The contract is between two people, not from one to the other and then maybe back again. This is at the core of the relationship between mother and infant, and when it is not created, must be rediscovered somewhere. Until then, a human being is partially present and more than partially in need of self-protection. This core is central to spiritual development, out of which esteem, safety, compassion, and response to others, develops. Missing it, we are amiss in our capacity to be fully human. Finding it, those parts of ourselves that were separated are returned to us, making us capable of wholeness. A colleague of mine referred to this as "blessing the trauma."

Once we land here in our work, the child conveys her story over and over in a relational field that tolerates the effects without moving away. The telling of the story is most often not in words per se, but in embodiment, metaphor, images in the tray, pictures drawn without any interpretation. The language of imagination and mending does not arise from the thinking brain. When a child's story is metaphorically revealed and understood long enough, she will begin to metabolize their experiences.

Mona's threat to me of swallowing unsafe plastic applies here. Her use of food had been both a body memory and a metaphor of survival. Her graphic vomiting was her body's experience of toxic neglect coming up and her own aggression. The behavior and the metaphor were united in their power. Someone needed to know what to do with all this ugliness.

Mona: The Wounds of Abandonment

Trust enters and begins its rebuilding. The child's story moves along, bringing in new characters and new realized effects, as if we are feeling through the old wounds from a variety of perspectives. At times it seems we are stuck, repeating the themes and images over and over. During these times, it is the therapist's task to add a bit of stress, a concern about one of the characters or something that returns the child to a felt relationship with the images and figures. As the child unwinds his story, there are times when implicit memory steps in and strongly reacts with a danger signal that we have not seen. We are in our belief that the child is chugging along, forward moving. It may become more difficult to see stuck moments when we are feeling relief that movement has been continual. It is imperative that we move with the child's pace, adding some pressure at times, being the memory's spokesperson who bridges yesterday and the future's hope into the moments of relationship in the room.

When child/therapist experiences have reclaimed a certain level of meaning, feelings connect or wire-up with thoughts and images. The pathway here is first of all the trust in the therapist and the child's capacity to depend on this guide. With that reliance in place, the child turns toward his own truths, which he believes will be understood. Mona's truths were open and vulnerable when she asked me if I would go all the way to China to find a baby. Would I find her?

Now the child is ready for symbolic integration of his experiences. Work with images, work that includes sandtray, art and movement, all assist in invoking images that assist in healing. The therapist is the receptive entity who can be trusted most of the time, who agrees to go together with the child to those places that intimacy works to avoid. Because it is the images that carry and contain the relationship, and these images are now playing out more organized stories from the child's self, the therapist is less a threat or an interference. The therapist has earned his spot as a representative, where two people can now be alone together. This is the third space where trust learns about itself, where the child might check out reality in the eyes of the therapist and find that, after 20 minutes, it is *still* safe, and still not scary.

Mona had shown me her terror of relying on an adult's care in her behaviors around apple cutting, and with her vomit. These entries into Mona's rage kicked off a series of oscillating (e.g., present/not present, calm/snarly) states, which seemed to enact her own helplessness of earlier pre-verbal experiences. Many times we entered pre-symbolic states, states that had not developed into safe relationship. Mona and I often played "concentration," a game of matching opposite feelings. Her stamina to identify her feelings in any words was very fragile. And yet, her desire to have matching cards on her side of the floor pushed her on. There were times that the cards were thrown at me. My task remained bringing calm back toward that flooded state before making any moves to rectify the situation.

Theories attempt to understand this place of swinging feelings, back and forth in their attempts to find center. They are entirely difficult to express without the work doing the telling. Mona was creating—discovering—a potential for mutuality by returning to the space that had not recognized her. When that emptiness entered the room, I often longed to leave myself, find something to distract the awful "visitors" from within her. Even getting up and getting a Kleenex could have convinced her I was not up for the ugly visitors. Going to this infant nonverbal place has the presence of raw matter, of twisting forms that simply just hurt. What Mona had accomplished was bringing forth the intolerable, just long enough for that to be seen before it might scamper off again. For her the intolerable was also *her*, a self that, through her "intolerable" gestures toward me, were communicated. Our body sensations got translated into psychic substance, which made that raw matter potentially useable, or capable of digestion.

The Child's Interior Map

What is this map that we follow into the child's needs and haunts and hurts? In any of the myriad of feelings that human beings have and that we share, it is of the essence that we are heard, understood and remembered. Using those essential requirements, our first act is to hear the child through the child's mode of speaking to us. Often times in therapy, that mode has been behaviors. The adults in the child's life, out of worry, efficiency, a desire to help the child learn society's rules, will want us to extinguish the behaviors that disturb them. Our own task, however, is to listen carefully and curiously for the child's vocabulary. I recall sitting with a 12-year-old, Luke, who had been suspended from school for carrying an illegal substance. He would not speak to anyone about his "problem." As miserable as we were together, we sat. Eventually he quietly told me, "Do you realize my family is a family of the abused? My mother has always been hit, two of my sisters, my grandma, my brother and me. We are the tribe of the hit." I felt the air go away, and we sat together some more, drawing a circle around his understanding. His risky behavior of carrying an illegal substance to school had yelled loudly, "Help me out! Get me out of here! I will do what it takes to break this inheritance." He had tried other methods of being heard, including getting his sister into a relative's home for protection. He resorted to a concrete "catch me, so I can speak." The "behavior problem" had been successful for him. He had finally found a way to bring publicity and some light to a very darkened landscape. First he had to find a way to be heard. Then we would need to find the tools with which we might build trust to use what we heard from this child, to weather the storms that come from the child's disbelief that we are willing to walk the walk of his experiences. And while we are walking, we create honest means to help the child understand that we remember that child and what is important, what language is being used. We are focused on decoding the language of behaviors in order to help the child bring order to his experiences.

The child's story is just that: this individual child's story. It is meant to make sense to this child. Sense-making carries subjectivity, a dot-to-dot image that reveals itself each time a new line is drawn to another dot, another meaning. The story Luke held was of intergenerational abuse, an assumed legacy whose burden overwhelmed him. Luke did not attempt change in this inheritance of sorts until he witnessed his own sibling in its grip. There seemed to be no one to hear his story of a clan that tacitly agreed to abuse. Luke stepped outside the private family collusions to create an intervention that might break open the story itself. Children make use of their behaviors in this way, in order to remain congruent with their own internal knowing. While they may be deeply troubled by the stories they see their adults acting upon, they themselves are not defended internally enough to ignore the tensions they experience between authenticity and emotional conflict. In this dissonance, children feel unheard and unseen. They frequently blame themselves, which adds pressure to finding a solution to the internal conflict.

Conflict between adult responses to a child's behavioral solutions can offer little relief. Many of our adult versions of problem-solving are in themselves justified. Our solutions, such as the DSM, are our best efforts to create procedures that organize our many questions around mental health. However, these same procedural efforts cannot overshadow the child's own story.

Therapeutic Tension

At times I allowed my attention to imagine the felt space between Mona and me as a single image. Together we were like an unpredictable tension before a storm, and at times the storm hailed down. Mona must try over and over to re-invent something or someone that otherwise had no concrete image. She had long ago lost the face and the memory of a birth mother. She reinvented pieces, stopped to grieve, accused me of causing the hurt she must address, and then went on digesting this messiness. This is where the psyche is perhaps the only force field strong enough, the only ground holy enough, upon which to lay this need.

Still later, Mona approaches meaning for the interior experience of having two mommies, her birth mom and her adoptive mom. In this, she is the birth parent and the parent/child connection of now. I am initially identified as the child over whom she has control. She packs a box of toys from the toy room, and we take a trip to visit my new family (in the bathroom, an appropriate spot for this memory). First I am the new mom, then I am just as quickly the child with two moms. Here the oscillations are outside of Mona and inside the relationship. This is a crucial step in healing and tolerating more intimacy. I decide to embody this tension and speak up, saying I only want one mommy. Mona goes into a tirade: "I need time with my husband! You follow me all over! You can have two mommies (is one daughter too much for one mom?)!"

I maintain my point, saying I want just one mommy. She tells me I am grumpy. I agree: "I'm grumpy, and it scares me when mamas yell like that."

Mona calms down, brings me pretend food. Then she sits peacefully and accepts real food from me: a sliced apple and a fruit bar. The person "outside" who has visited her person "inside" comes back together, and I am a safe nurturer who can do some things right. Even sharing in the tension of mother/child, I am somewhat trustworthy. Mona's implicit memories are now capable of refreshing themselves within this mutual experience of fast-changing identities and responses.

Transference engages the child's trust that it is safe to recover dependency. In its recovery, the child rediscovers the original map that returns her to where she was hurt, where the fragments still wait to be found and fitted together again. The therapist here is a midwife, the close-at-hand presence whose reckonings of the child's truths enable the child to integrate such thoroughly unconcrete aspects of self. The therapist accepts the child's stories as emotionally valid, with all the ins and outs and worries of that dancing, as a mother had originally meant to do and be. In this relationship of renewed trust, the child pulls together his own feelings, thoughts, and interior forces, investing them with the name of his own. With the therapist as active witness, the child and the child's own internal wisdom mend the original map that belongs to this one child alone. Herein lies the response to the question so often asked: "Will you remember me?"

Mona imagined her own map of healing through metaphor that sustained accurate descriptions of her experiences of abandonment. Attending to her descriptions together brought her isolated internal processes into expressions that she could tolerate. Mona and I had practiced a back-and-forth role-playing that is about much more than roles. Our play contained the inner voices that, if left unheard by another, become the dictators to self fragments in adults. In Mona's play, her own map of resilience acted toward the hope we carried together. It became evident to me that as we worked together, Mona's behaviors, which were very difficult for her adoptive parents to cope with, were the staying power of an innate strength that kept Mona believing in her own potential relationship.

Part III

Working in Transference: The Use of the Therapist

CHAPTER 10

Marnie: Co-transference

"Play is something we do together—in an ongoing dyadic *movement*. In its broadest sense, play is movement, a back and forth between us, that has its own direction or contour which both partners shape and surrender to" (Benjamin, 2018).

We can unpack some of the words that Benjamin succinctly uses. In "both partners shape and surrender to..." the word *both* points out that two people attend in this process. Surrendering to rhythmicity has a number of meanings: "to give up in favor of another"; "to give over to something"; "to relinquish possession or control of to another because of demand or compulsion." And the word rhythmicity is important, too: to flow back and forth in cadence, together. These are worded approaches that initiate our own loosening, our own efforts to understand what transference and co-transference is. It underlines the engagement of two, with no lineation.

Co-transference is doing and being together. To separate transference into two pathways, transference and counter-transference, implies that two separate dynamics are ensuing. This is partially true. The addition to this truth is that these two dynamics have joined forces. The back-and-forth movement between child and therapist establishes its own harmony. To go there, we are required to give up our definitions and our diagnoses in favor of another and that other person's meanings. When we are embedded in the mutual space of this other, we will suffer the effects of transference. This is the field of co-transference, the "thirdness," where we enter into relationship as a "participant from the inside out" (Benjamin, 2018). From inside, we learn of the child from the child. We will submit our knowledge of the child's history to the child's own perceptions of events, in order to find out, to know from a mutual viewpoint of that "us" that Zack worked from. In doing so, we surrender to the child's story, sustained in implicit memory. We therapists accept the paradox of being both inside the child's metaphors, and holding a containment that utterly belongs to the child's own authentic self. There will be time later in the therapy to update that story by integrating current experiences into that story.

The Back and Forth of Co-transference

In play therapy, the doorway into this thirdness, or "usness" is through metaphor that carries in its images the child's subject-feelings. The feelings may well be initially chaotic and disorganized, waiting to be funneled into the witness's comprehension. Remember that implicit memory jostles its way into implicit reality, right now, right here in this play. We are within shared space that will eventually make use of our adult capacity to rotate feeling states into words. But in the moment, with the child, we have entered as that guest, to learn about something together that neither of us has uncovered before.

It is up to the therapist to make possible this participation, through playthings that are available within an enclosed safe space. The child (not the therapist) brings feeling states into this relationship for further understanding. The therapist holds and tends to the relationship that is being established within the child's inner environment. The child must feel safe and witnessed in order to reveal his inner meanings. As his meanings come into the room through play, through an imaginative world that includes the child's experiences, the therapist continues to receive, to relate with the child's inner world. This is a step further than to relate *to*. We are certain enough of the child's authentic truths that we will go with the child in search of those truths and of any shrapnel that may be caught in the experiences of them, imagining with the child what this inner world carries. The therapist's own thoughts are not the fabric of the child's imagination that is carrying us toward the unseen past.

The child's own understandings serve as the deep supply of material that is being brought forth. The great challenge in going with the child to these shared spaces is that we will encounter along with the child what feeling states are stored in that reservoir. We will touch the child's own experiences that have remained unconscious and undigested if they have been perceived as too dangerous. Other times we will feel what happened, making emotional contact with the one who created the breakage. In these joined states, we are both our own trained professional selves and the affective feelings the child has transferred into our relationship.

We circle straight back into the more "primitive" feeling states: those states that had too little shared empathy and were therefore left out, left in implicit memory as unknown because they were frightening. At these junctures we become the mothering principle that cradles those states in order that they may be found, slowly digested, and made visible enough for repair. Relating-with is about this back-and-forth cadence of the infant/mother. To be clear, we are not approaching the child as an infant, and surely we are no mother replacement. We simply undertake the profound dynamics of "standing by" in reliable availability, toward this child's own memory-meanings, believing in the child's own authorship of her felt history. Through all this effort, this deep labor into relationship, the therapist is simply not in control of changing the child's implicit memory. Even to approach this may cause a renewed effort on the part of the child to be invisible, to try not to be hurt again.

In the prior chapter, Mona threw her pain out into the room without mercy. Once she felt my presence in her experiences, she made use of "my" badness, "my" unwillingness to be with her as a baby. And yet, clearly this abandonment was not one I had been present to. In a real sense, the badness was "ours," and together we searched for a solution to this hurt. She was demanding that I be present *now*, climb into a missing piece and experience its loss and rage. As these unloved and therefore unlovable parts entered our shared space, several dynamics needed to be present at once. I needed to embody the danger without being dangerous. I needed to soothe myself as I experienced being that danger of her past, while making every attempt to sense the feelings she threw into me. The feelings of rage also contained such deep misery. I felt the unresolved wailing of the infant, the anger and Mona's own belief that I would do what had already been done. At times I wanted to stick up for myself and leave this misery. I wanted to put some sort of reality in this container, that I was safe, that I would not hurt her. I wanted to take care of myself out loud, interrupting the narration of her pain by saying it was not mine. And yet, in order to endure the space from which Mona herself would surrender to being lovable, I needed to continue to own, re-own, and own again my reactive states. I needed to stay awake. By maintaining a kind of reverie state rather than a thinking state, I could name the relationship presence in the room, my own need to make distance, and then the place in which to have no distance.

Mona contained such fierceness in her personality, an innate gift that was difficult to tolerate. She carried so much of the pathway to her own mending. Her gestures of peeing on me and of vomiting on me brought up my own abandonment. I did not appreciate those ghost visits, and wanted to scurry away like a tiny insect, away from her barrage. At the very same time, I experienced a deep respect for her, feeling a survivor at hand that coerced me into seeing. Mona's strength of self was wound up within her pain. As we clumsily found one another through these rhythmic mergings and separations, my respect grew. This feeling of respect assisted me in hearing the both of us bundled together in one burden in her play. Mona had not been carried, and she was pushing me with her own experiences of being too big a burden to be carried. Many times, all I could muster in the moment was to stay in place, with all our mutual states arguing there in the play, a small boat in a big current. It was my responsibility to carry the both of us and the mutual space where we resonated.

Feeling the Mutual "Us" Space

The therapist might feel the feelings that the child cannot yet have. The behaviors and the feelings are two roads and the therapist straddles them, as the child accesses behaviors as a relief from the feelings. Play therapists often will mistake their work as helping the child to become aware of their behaviors. If behaviors are the outward signs of inner turmoil, and these signs take up our attention, the turmoil itself has little to no room to emerge. The therapist has gotten caught in a form of logic: this child will do better when an adult, "me," can bring light to the behaviors. Very little light enters when the driver of actions is not seen. And not being seen, the child continues to pull up her sense of a worthless self with its meanings of sadness, losses, and shame.

Implicit memory is unconscious. And yet it carries what all of us have pieced together and placed there. Children who suffer from trauma contain these memories without a caring other to honor what they "know" happened. The recorded patterns of an early self live in the feeling and perceiving self. Neurons that direct behaviors are not the behaviors themselves. These early patterns are who we are and they drive how we approach others. The task of the play therapist is to find sparks in these patterns and to track those sparks. We might say that the therapist pulls together these sparks simply by perceiving them. From this collection a fire begins, and the fire burns the old until there is room for something new. This is the myth of the phoenix rising from the ashes. It is not the therapist's task to be the phoenix, nor to create ash for this transformational image to emerge. The therapist and the child are together bringing what has not been containable into the mind, where very early patterns transform as they are carried along.

The Dangers of Transference Work

We therapists need to understand the depth and danger of the transference state, to both our clients and ourselves. Transference is not a sacred goal to be reached by the wizened therapist. We are not protected from its turmoil simply because we can address its presence academically. To find ourselves in that domain, we need to know about its landscape because, once in it, ignorance will be the primary reason for mistakes. Transference requires that we understand why our clients will not go toward this confluence of an "us." Many times the client will use dissociation to remain outside the empathic pull that would lead to transference. Trust the client. It is likely that there still is not enough muscle or stamina to stretch into the risk of relationship. Our task becomes building the stamina and relational trust that will allow us to move closer. For a person who has not learned to dance, and may in fact have the experience that dancing was dangerously dizzying, the trustworthiness of rapport and bending into mutual fields can be too disorienting. The first step, then, is to understand the child's own inner landscape and attend to those signals (chaotic trays, overbearing bossiness, inability to dialogue in any fashion) that tell us not to come too close just yet.

By obeying the child's pacing, we are in fact allowing the child to come closer. We are not avoiding close encounters, but rather, building the roadways into wiring-up more deeply. This effort goes against most adult expectations that want to bring the child to better behaviors. "Better" is fair warning: better for whom? The child must have reason to avoid relational trust until such time as he leans toward the therapist. Most commonly, these experiences of trust will create triggers of the past experiences that become located in our present. If the child is not ready for that past undigested material to erupt into our therapeutic space and the intimacy of the trust, then enactment is bound to follow unreadiness.

One of my first child clients taught me about this. He was 5 years old when we started. His parents were intensely eager that Eli and I address his experiences of molestation. I keenly felt the parents' anxiety and my empathy went to them. I was able to sort out Eli's experiences with him, but after leaving my office Eli went to pre-school and immediately acted out his experiences with another child. That was on my watch, regardless of my not being in the school. I had worked too quickly, arousing feelings that had their context, their implicit reality. I had not listened to the child's own pace. His experience had come to the forefront through behaviors, while I had not yet found what he needed me to understand. I worked this failure in myself for some time in order to understand the differences between the child's needs and the parents' needs and where my own new-therapist self had engaged in overstepping this child's pace. I needed to work with the parents to help them with their containment as I worked with Eli and his right-brain meanings.

The "Remote Control" Metaphor

I begin seeing Marnie when she is halfway between 3 and 4 years old. Marnie has spent her young life with a very addicted mom and a series of "dads." She is referred to me through our Sexual Assault Program. She is feisty and at the same time loveable and charming. Marnie approaches me bravely, with eye contact and a need for conversation. At the same time, I detect a distance that she herself controls. I feel intrusive when I come too close. Her verbal invitations are full of questions about me. She immediately seems hungry for some reflection of who she might be, as if she has not fully become a separate self and is assigning me that task.

In the first few weeks, Marnie might approach what she senses is profound pain, and then suddenly her arm shoots out toward me and she aggressively states, "I'm turning you off now. No more talking! No more!" What she holds invisibly in her hand that points directly at me is a remote control for a T.V. When this happens, I sort of gasp and put my hand over my mouth, muttering "No more!" If I disobey, she comes closer and with her arm nearly at my mouth, clicking away, she shouts, "Off!" I learn to obey this need to control what could and could not yet be felt between us.

The invisible control mechanism kept both Marnie and me out of reach of the unspeakable. Marnie's imagination was itself unable to envision a way through her day-to-day helplessness. Marnie's resiliency held her in place, and held my thoughts at bay. Before she could open up the possibility of something new, something as yet unimagined by her, she first needed to control reality and be sure I could stick with that need. It was Marnie's body that sensed trouble. It was her body's alertness that clicked at me when I moved too close to the vigilance she held in place. I think it was the remote control that ignited our transference. The sudden aggression from such a little body, shooting invisible but deadly rays at me to STOP! put me in front of her need. Sidestepping this urgent gesture would have been too painful for her. Others had already done that to her body. I was the layer of "skin" that provided her with some slow remembering of her self as a separate human being, with a movement that stopped me from broaching this too quickly. In the moment I could not have elaborated on this. I simply experienced "STOP" in my body, as if coming any closer was just wrong.

Marnie takes to the toys as states of her own neediness. She also loves to paint and makes large splotches of blue, black, and red. At first her mess-making frightens her. But as she watches me carefully for response and reaction, and finds that I appear to enjoy her messiness, Marnie becomes more expressive with paints. She often delights in painting her hands and mine, finding that this makes us somehow more "alike." We wash up together, dry our hands and arms together, with a charged arena in our close proximity. During some of these times, Marnie calls me Mama and looks at me, confused. I am fully aware that Marnie has inserted me as her surrogate mother, and I am cautious to both keep my boundary of her need present and keep her felt sense of requiring a mothering energy present. What I am not as aware of is that Marnie is also sharing the sensate invasions she had experienced.

Therapeutic "Failure"

This play within dualities with Marnie is difficult. It pushes upon us to be actively in love with our little clients, while containing the limits of what and who we cannot become. And what we can and cannot do.

Marnie's first extended play theme, while she continues to remote control our environment, is of being a child that had gotten lost in the woods. She takes a plaid blanket and lays it behind the rocking chair, which becomes the door into my "house." (The metaphor of a rocking chair being a gateway is so beautiful: the often-used chair for lullabies and rest. In Marnie's work it is surely an empty rocker.) She lets me know that there are scary animals where she stays, out there in the woods. I myself feel her fear, and I hate that I am safely inside. This deep agitation in me is what works in me to fail Marnie. She knocks on the back of the rocking chair/door and says she is cold. I immediately ask if she wants to come in and warm up. She looks at me with a sort of resignation or pity and says no.

Marnie had gotten deeply into my own heart. She was so present and yet so unwilling to be seen, like an animal in the woods who darts in and out of the shadows but never leaves. You always know it is watching you, and you grow more impatient, perhaps, to know who this is who continues to evade you. Marnie's circumstances were familiar to me. In addition to her work in my office, Marnie's mother was working with a gifted therapist, and we had a signed release to share what this twosome was asking for and what resources were needed. Looking back, my own admiration for this other therapist also pushed me on. I wanted to see change and safety.

Once Marnie believed me enough, her imagination moved closer to her need. Becoming a child lost in the woods became her own story. It traveled us both toward her, toward where she was lost. Her resilience continued to pace me, not allowing me to trespass what she needed me to hear. When I had not heard well enough, we had to start over, like being in a game where you have to go back to the beginning because you selected the wrong card. Except that my cards were my own dismal handicaps. The transference worked within me. It let me know that I could not manage her pain yet. I had to turn back to the place in the journey where I had dropped the "us" between us and began running desperately for some solution. I had no desire to leave Marnie in her deserted and intruded body. I could not find the match there, and I did not know where I was failing.

In the first session of this interaction, Marnie simply gets more and more upset. I become more determined. I want to see that I

Marnie: Co-transference

am "doing it right," and Marnie's facial responses to my efforts do not communicate that. In the second session of this experience, she again sets up the blanket and again tells me she is cold. She adds that she is hungry. I don't know if I catch on in this session or the next. I do have in my notes that I felt desperate. Because of therapeutic team work, I know her mom is still using and still being abused. As far as I can tell, nothing is happening that connects me to those identified "issues." Marnie is simply refusing to come in from the cold! As Marnie leans toward relational trustworthiness, I run ahead of her and internally insist, "I am here! Just a little to your right and we will connect!" My impatience is driven by my deep worry for Marnie. I want Marnie to land in something safe: me. A great mistake on my part.

But something, at some delayed point, becomes conscious in me: my own anxiety, my deep worry for her, all the resources I have that are not on the other side of the rocking chair/door. With a deep sense of grief and resignation, I keep the "door" open and ask Marnie if she has a bed. "Sort of." Does she have any food? "No." Would she let me get some from my kitchen and send it out to her? "Yeah." We are getting somewhere, while internally I want to grab her and force her to come inside. I simplistically tell Marnie that I wish she could come in but that she cannot because I might be a danger. I go over to the dollhouse and make a plate of toy food, bring it over and hand it through the door. She thanks me and "closes the door." I manage this door clicking shut. She knows deep inside that I had accepted the transfer of her neediness.

As Marnie continued to rely on this "us," she continued to turn back when I failed. She educated me. Where we had to go did not allow my savior efforts. Marnie trusted me enough to build the vessel she needed, one into which we both fit tight. Once she knew in her body that I would not step into her space, she taught me where to move to find her. All of this back and forth remained unconscious. I was the one who needed to bring some recognition to where the crisis lived. She used the transference to expose me to myself so that I became conscious of her pain in me. She waited me out. The more I was able to recognize how lost she was, the closer she came. This interchange held us both. I did not like it, although I loved Marnie. Her determination was honorable. Imagine the journey all the way back to the mother's body. She got all the way there, and then, very chaotically, started the process of developing into a separate self. We held that separateness together, too.

This control from Marnie over what she could accept from me hurts me. At the same time, she is teaching me what it takes for trust to grow. Trust has little to do with rescue and everything to do with walking together through the swampy morass of felt experiences. That is what we have here: her story, a felt, disorganized, labyrinth of experiences with little witnessing or remembering of Marnie herself. She insists that we go together to where she might explore her own perceptions.

Our time together moves more deeply into images that are hard to bear and need not be named here. Marnie puts aside those remote-control buttons once I understand what might happen if she comes through the door. Eventually Marnie does come "inside" and sits with her blanket in her lap, willing to eat a cereal bar in my presence.

Two or three steps in Marnie's process are worth naming here. She paints very simple streaks of blue across a paper, and with delight, makes a "person." In the water she puts some blue dots. "These are sharks," she tells me. "It's ok—this person swims here." Her smile betrays the gap between her story and the danger she has painted. Although I am able to narrate her story back to her, I add that it is not ok because sharks are dangerous, and she ignores me. The difference between reality and her show of feelings makes my body ache. Her reality is that it seems ok to "swim with sharks." Marnie still needs to believe that her mother is keeping her safe, and she remains oftentimes numb to how unsafe she feels but cannot yet address. I step backward and make every effort to build the steppingstones that might slowly decrease this gap. Meanwhile, Marnie's own clash between a need to be seen and a numbness of feeling pushes my efforts to bring her to a congruent place in feelings.

Reliance on the Child's Pace

Marnie remained determined to teach me this: that there was to be no getting ahead of her own capacity to trust and rely on me. This speaks volumes to the child's rights, the child's own center and frame of reference. It is not our task to shift this center. It is our task to learn from the child what is wounded or diminished or off-center. The child longs for someone to know about this off-center state. The frame of reference required for this center to be findable lies in the relationship, in the dependence of the child, and on the guidance of the parent. And in therapy, the child must feel found and discovered in order to choose to bend toward the "surrogate parent."

One reason we are so alarmed to be a surrogate is because many of us have been told that the child needs to make these steps toward the parent right off the bat. When a child has suffered, perhaps not at the hands of these parents but another set who are now gone from the child's life, that child needs a "remote control" to govern *any* one coming yet again into that wounded space. After all, an adult was clumsy; I am an adult; therefore I will be clumsy. This goes for the adopting parent, too. Distress from such emotional ineptness has resulted in trauma. If the child perceives more of the old stress, he will not approach. We are offering recognition of this old experience while we hold out with something unknown to the child, something approaching stamina that remains steady within the child's explorations. The therapist will be the transitional figure who assists the child in building trust in order to reach out to an available foster or adoptive parent. It is as if a template must be built, an architecture of trust, prior to trying trust out on yet another parent who the child must rely on for survival. For survival, yes, but for healing, maybe not. The therapeutic, relational template is the transitional bridge into trust. There is simply no magic that allows the fiction that since I chose you, little one, I am certain you will also choose me. The remote control becomes the defense mechanism that keeps the clumsy adult from being overly blundering and making past pain occur right here, right now.

Where Marnie needs to be found, ultimately, is in her newborn and pre-born self. Using all her courage and an eruption of overwhelming feelings, she drives us both back to a mama carrying a baby in her "tummy." She puts this mama in a hospital bed near my chair. Marnie expresses helplessness, neediness, anger, and despair as she frantically tries to create a concrete image of the baby outside the mama going back inside the mama. I slow my breathing down, attempting to walk with both of us toward this new, unborn image. I feel a kind of numbness that tells me I can easily solve this. And I hear myself thinking that, and step back as if I am under water.

With my offer, she agrees to put the baby under the bed and know it is inside. She narrates that this new baby would come out and maybe be a good baby. I hear the commentary behind this: "I have been a bad baby. I could not make a safe mama. Maybe this time, I can be the right kind of baby."

After this most challenging work together, Marnie relaxes into the changes she chooses to make. She is often very angry at her mother, who has quit using and is struggling to take on a little girl who has found she wants a mother. Work continues, with Marnie's strengths becoming more her own, and with her mother's attempts at building personal strength.

So this was Marnie's perception: in that centering frame of reference, she believed she could do something other than her implicit experiences mirrored within her that would protect Mama from all the pain the two of them shared in their fused space. As this space in therapy found some separateness on behalf of her, Marnie revealed her own sense of profound responsibility toward her mother. It was not that Marnie was unloved. It was that she had not been seen developmentally as a separate self coming into being. Without this ability to be loved while separating, the child's center continues on in the assumption of being the parent's witness rather than reveling in the joy of being witnessed. Marnie could not find herself in her story.

Neither of us would have done well in a mutual transference as long as Marnie was so merged with her mother's pain and her mother's choices around lack of safety. It was Marnie who stayed in the wilderness in a corner of the playroom until I could muster the strength to see her private experience. I had to become the inability to help, to separate. I would need to offer something new that neither of us would know once I stopped offering fused anxiety. Somehow, with the rocking chair being our barrier, both the harm done and the hope of mending stood together. Benjamin identifies this as *meta-communication.* "Meta-communication is this: a form of reflecting or creating difference without disrupting rhythmicity, staying inside the flow rather than stepping outside to comment, performing recognition in action" (Benjamin, 2018).

My own triggers lie deep in the place of lack of recognition in some periods of intrusive pain in my own family of origin. I was stumbling as Marnie's work found a fragile time in my own younger history that had occurred at about the same age she was. I would have to do more personal work, and bring a renewed courage to my own implicit memories, as I held on while Marnie brought her resilience into play between us. She did, however, build the courage to go back to where she had lost her self's center and begin to build that precious frame of reference that finds one's self good, worthy, and loveable.

In this state of co-occupancy, the therapist is charged with holding the child's implicit memories as they become current again. They are current in the relationship and being played in the toys. They are not verbal, although verbal communication can take place. The therapist holds the electric current, that current that is reaching to trust an adult, again, as it makes a new effort to be felt and acted upon in the therapy setting, and in the relationship of trustworthiness. This is the healing joint. When the therapist has made contact with her own old harms and has attended to them in herself, she is a more worthy container that truly offers the safety that could not be offered without her own self-awareness. That self-awareness shoulders a private pain and lets it remain off-stage while the real work is on-stage, within the child's own urgent healing.

CHAPTER 11

Jake: Building the Self

Jake enters his first session seeming very guarded. His first request is "Do you have an uncurled snake?" I do, but he does not play with this. He gathers a group of cows and names each one as a family member. "For you," he says, as he puts in "wild animals: a buffalo, a hyena, a tiger." He identifies himself already in this first tray as the saber-toothed tiger. I am to hold on to the untamed wildness, that, more than any other family member, represents Jake himself. Family members are not defined in these characters: they are simply "family."

With some effort, he then identifies himself as the Hunter. "I couldn't wish to be a Hunter. The single animals hide from the Hunter." One definition of hunter is: "one who searches for or seeks something: a treasure hunter."

Still approaching his trust in me, Jake puts two knights in the tray. "Are these two on the same team?" (Me: "Are they?") "Oh yes. They are. One is a king. One is a queen." Then there are a lot of fighting noises, where guards are added and stumble and tumble about in the sand. Jake identifies himself as the king and queen. "There's only one left of yours. But I got pretty much alive." This is my entry into the dynamics. I am already slipping into the overwhelming aspect of feelings that Jake carries. He lets me know that I am not doing so well, although Jake is "coming alive." I wonder what I am meant to carry; some sort of burden that has ache in it, certainly someone who "is not doing so well."

Finding the Primitive Self through Image

This child, Jake, will help both him and me find the images that speak of his leadership in this process. This will be a long portrayal of a child's process in order to reveal the depths of where children often go in their "primitive" selves: their "self-taught artistry." To be here, in this child's process, wondering what the child wants to let me know today, I must let go of my own preoccupation with myself, with the diagnosis the child carries, and with my concern that I have to help this child be less (fill in the blank) or more (fill in the blank). And fair warning: to stay with Jake's work is to feel as if we are caught as a big fish is caught. A large hook has impaled itself in our logic, and we are struggling to free ourselves and return to the world of known sympathy and support for a little person who is in this degree of felt discomfort. At the same time, Jake himself would not allow that kind of dismissal of his need. He demanded that, once found, I stayed with him, swimming in the murky waters of not-known. He required that I stay until he could find himself. And in that, he is more like one of the old knights at the Round Table, agreeing to go on a hunt for the Grail. And I was often his horse, begging to go back to the barn! Big fish or old horse: these are my images that let me know Jake's thorough need of my presence.

Children approach their days with the same importance that adults do. Our ability to comprehend the depth of children has historically been profoundly hampered by the beliefs that children are adults in the making, waiting to grow up to claim their wholeness. In reality, children often have a close access to their truths, albeit in unexplored language. Their language is closer to the bone, close to what has been referred to as "primitive." That word, *primitive*, helps us out: "not derived from something else; relating or belonging to forces of nature; a self-taught artist." In its root, *primitive* points us to other meanings from the same root, such as *primal* and *primary*, which mean "first, foremost: he who takes first place; chief, leader, from former, original." Feelings are communicated in children's images and behaviors. These images are original, created by the "self-taught artist" within each child.

Linking this up with imagination, which is a child's own healthy engine of creativity, imagination is "the power of the mind to form images, especially of what is not present to the senses." I would add that imagination *enhances* what is available to the senses, expressing images from what is discovered within implicit reality. Imagination promotes a child's ability to "speak" from his own internal creative world. In attending to images, we are really making a second swipe at what we mean by primitive, prime, relating to the forces of nature. A child lives so close to this world. A clearer way to say this is that the child's life is still within the currents of this imaginative world, and she makes use of that embedded world in her language.

The Willingness of the Therapist

When we defend the absolute requirement that safe relationship must be present for imagination to emerge in play, the willingness of the therapist to stand by unconditionally enables the child to make use of this acceptance and trust his imagination as his spokesperson. The therapist is not the healer. He is the witness to this growing trust in the self of the child. The therapist understands that his position is "as ally and guide" within the child's own story and personal myth (Bernstein, 2005). Imagination rouses the child's own interior mythological world. With the full attention of the witness, the child trusts that powerful force that is created both from the child's personal world and from the felt sense of the child's meanings. This is the thing: in this moment, the therapist is present for this child and this child's efforts alone. And the child relies on this presence of another to trust herself to an interior world that is always available and had veiled itself or closed down for any number of reasons. "Relying" on someone: the word has come from "leig: to bind," which is "to have faith in," or to bind oneself to another in trust. It is so important to truly understand who we ourselves are in the work, and who we are in service to, in order to remain reliable—our skills within reach—to this powerful presence within the child. Our own openness brings us the gifts of the child's use of us. This is the meaning of the third space and of co-transference: the child, ourselves, and the unknown. This third space, the imaginal, governs healing. It cannot be emphasized enough: The child approaches this space of healing through the strength of the unconditional regard within the relationship when this regard has been built and is ready for use from the child's un-languaged and fully knowing vocabulary of self. It is really this "primitive" power, what is within and not conditioned by the constructs of a language-bearing grid, that children access. Trust finds the child.

Many parents and teachers call a therapist for support of a child because the child's behaviors are the symptoms calling for help. In therapy, some children more quickly re-organize what has been troubling them. Concerned behaviors diminish. This shorter-term play therapy has its place: perhaps parents have reorganized dynamics that were affecting the family system; the child was moved to a school environment that is more congruent with his needs; the symbols that the child has engaged in therapy have found their way in to the child's expressions. For some children, however, the relationship with the therapist serves as a bridge into the deeper dynamics within a child, such as warring internal battles between being loyal to Dad and suffering from that same dad's unpredictable aggressions. These deep opposing perceptions

Jake: Building the Self

and meanings will require the trust, perhaps even the love in the therapist, that will enable the child to feel along the recesses of these conflicts and find an enduring resolution. That resolve will not come from being given a solution of sorts by an outside voice. And the child is most capable of discovering and then demanding that the therapist be present in that hour, and that the tools and toys also be there in that hour, sealing the ordinary environment off from an otherwise logical belief that it is just a room with toys.

Imagination

Imagination is the linchpin that swivels us from compromising to the needs of the world around us to listening to a different voice that communicates from within, through the body and through imagining what the body and our internal communicator are saying (Ammann, 1991). There are, however, degrees, if you will, of imagination. I can say, "I imagine that…" and still be wired to my logic. Imagination at the depth of creating, however, offers a way to express an image that floats just a bit out of reach of the ability to talk about it. The environment has become somewhat alive. To imagine in this way, we jump into the image. We race with and morph into the metaphor. We are not simply listening for something to speak with us, but rather, we are engaged. Children have this jumping-in down pat. I'll never forget a 5-year-old who was beginning to read. We sat together reading a book all about the sound of long vowel *u*. When she came to the page about "blue," she stopped with a blissful look and said to me, "Blue… Isn't that the best color of all? Blue." We shared the fullness of blue for a bit. I felt the gift she opened to me, of blueness, deep inside. What a remarkable thing to have color-feelings. And further, to have blue surround two people together.

There is a paradox active right here: If I attempt to put language onto the child's forms of expression, the more veiled the resource

203

becomes. As imagination guides the child's work to deeper and deeper levels, a kind of fusion between feelings and toys takes place, which is at the heart of using sandtray and art. The feelings illuminated though the toys are deep emotions, which lessen both the use of and the need for words as communication.

Let's approach Jake and his work, and the power of his imagination. Jake had just turned 4 when we began his journeying together. He was very aggressive with his temper tantrums and would not or could not listen to what was expected of him. His home seemed to be stable and healthy. I would learn that this was a front that Jake had made it his task to kick down. His father was in and out of FEMA (Federal Emergency Management Agency) events. This unpredictable on-call reality and the seeming disappearance of Dad eroded this young child's efforts at stability. His dad often brought back home with him the traumas he himself had experienced in helping others through large crises such as hurricanes and fires. Unidentified and resistant in its presence, Jake's dad suffered from post-traumatic stress. His mom was suffering deeply under the strain of this marriage, with its emotional and verbal abuse. But none of this was given at the intake. I was in the dark, and so was Jake.

This hero has two sisters, and he is in the middle. Early on in his work, his parents separated and then divorced. Jake's own external reality of very conflicted parents made it so difficult to hold on to beliefs that his mom loved him when he was at Dad's, knowing Mom did not love Dad and was afraid of Dad's temper, and having a third "parent-like" adult, and then a fourth, come into his life. All these pieces had little understanding given to him. What they did have was a constant hodge-podge of unpredictable emotions, with one feeling conflicting with another within short periods of time, like shocks without shock absorbers. And during all this, Jake's development was attempting to stabilize a "me," while he was not sure who he belonged with, or who would be the vessel of some sort of "us" that merited his trust and dependence.

Jake's Internal War

I saw Jake for more than two years during this first round of work. I would see him again when his mother was hospitalized for a lengthy illness, during which time Jake lived the life of an orphan. As a lead in to this work, what Jake was able to reveal and then overcome involved two major themes that were fast becoming the myths he lived by: that his parents warred over him, and because of his sensitivities, he could not resolve the war; and that he believed that the war had really usurped the truth that he was loved. At the core of Jake's tantrums was a baby's voice of "Look at me... look at ME." This war seemed to take place in the arguments above him and inside his heart.

Jake is nearly panicky in his need to engage me as a carrier of what bothers him. This is often what happens. As the child gains trust, the therapist begins to carry the "problem" as the child perceives it. Jake feels his behaviors are the problem, and he is going to get my help in figuring out the awfulness of that belief. After all, his parents are at war with one another. Somewhere in the first 3 months I have been told that the parents may separate for some "peace of mind" for Mom. Dad tells Jake that he is heartbroken.

Within 2 months, Jake has grown strong enough to represent his vulnerable self with images in the tray. "Do you have a baby (rhinoceros)? Jake needs to be between the mommy and daddy, cuz he's so little." Is Jake telling me that such a little entity needs protection, or is he too small to come between Mom and Dad? He offers some clue when he says, "The turtle is slow because he has a load in him." At that point he states, "My mommy got upset at my daddy. Actually, my mommy or daddy didn't get upset. Weird mommy! Weird daddy!" Jake's understanding of the fighting comes out and then is too frightening in its constellation of words. Possibly, to identify parents warring at this stage of Jake's work simultaneously names him as the bad guy, the fighter. In their focus on self, children often identify themselves as the one causing the problem and being the problem. Nonetheless, Jake hangs on to having said his truth. I am certain that he scans me to see if I need to change his initiating definition of "war."

Another of Jake's themes with its images was of being the family pet. At times in his sand stories this pet was left out of family activities and family rituals, and in these times that pet was penned. Other times this pet was able to express Jake's anger through his bizarre behaviors. The pet became very mean, and Jake himself would scamper between images in his effort to let the images speak while being quite afraid of what they might reveal.

"I'm this powerful animal! I'm strong! I could kill this other tiger. I could knock this fence (a penned area) down. I'm the guy's pet." (There is a sense of good and bad having no stability at all. I'm anxious.)

"Guys throw food onto the tiger. He's real mad now! Two guys fight me. ('He' has shifted to 'I' now.) They're fighting over their home. I don't have any blood. I'm the only bad animal. All the other animals are good animals. Except me. I'm bad." (I had discovered that in more pressing tantrums, Jake would throw his plate of food during a meal.)

After this, Jake initiates aggression in the tray, using animals that he states are brave, powerful, and aggressive. He brings his siblings in through the naming of various animals, and gleefully lets me know that he himself is the strongest and can win any fight. He can make himself become more than one animal, too. He has become more agitated, angry with me, frustrated that the toys are being played with by others and removed from their known places. Jake is depending more and more on these "toys" to be *alive, to be where he can find them because they carry who he is feeling himself to be.*

The Toys as Alive Feeling States

This transference into the toys is crucial to understand when it happens. Kids ask that toys be moved into hiding. They may attempt to put them in their pockets and take them home, for the sake of those toys not being lost. The child cannot afford to have something happen to the toys, toys that have become parts of themselves. These toys/images/feelings have become capable of making a new kind of sense inside of the child. It would then be tragic if a toy goes missing during the time in which it belongs to the child's interior sort of mapmaking world.

During this time Jake's theme was one of the powerful sabertooth tiger collapsing into one of the family pets. Jake approached a deep depression as his false courage weakened. Perhaps Jake had had to separate too early from parent protection. When this occurs, a false independence, a bravado, takes place during developmental windows that would otherwise call upon some separation, and yet would remain tucked in to the parent attachment. In his play he expressed anger and frustration when the tiger's power went unnoticed by other miniature family representatives. And in his environment, Jake expressed the deep difficulty of being as "strong" as he wanted himself to be. This effort often broke loose in aggressive behaviors, both at home and in the playroom.

Because I knew more of the family history by now, and the blunt comings and goings of Dad, I could embody and make more sense of Jake's frustrations. I knew we were working together on something unnamable at this point, and I seemed to become a participant through the voices my body whispered. During this building phase, more often than not my own sensations expressed themselves in my head in the self-talk of frustration that I did not know enough, that someone else would have made a better witness than myself, that I had no assistance available for Jake. I risked these voices being part of the shared space rather than being my own truth, separate from the work that had encircled us both. Separating these whispers into mental truths would have separated my ability to trust Jake and to follow his lead. I needed to nod to the voices while not giving in to them.

Jake continued on with a ferocious kind of energy. I suspected that this furor was the same that had demanded the attention he sorely needed, and now it was constellating in a safer way for him to better organize around his own needs. Parents reported that his tantrums were calming, and they were surprised and pleased. But I knew Jake had only just begun, particularly because of the "pet" theme that was making so much meaning for him.

Jake continues to suffer the experiences of the bad and powerful animals. He purposely uses physical distance between the animals as his own physiological relief from the tensions of acting upon his internal definition of the bad guy. At some point Jake includes me in this physical experiment, telling me when I am too close and then asking that I be very close. We are in labor together, trying to find out how to comfort this little boy's sensitive feelings and confusing aggressions. Too close; too far away– these are the unstable contractions of suffering.

During this time, in his play his toy family members seemed to become less confusing and less powerful for Jake. His own aggression was figuring out how to be helpful to him as a communicator, rather than isolating him. As he worked me in this push/pull dynamic, he seemed like a 2-year-old who demands that the world is his oyster and anyone in that world of oyster pearl-making needs to listen! I was certainly falling deeper into connection with Jake, wondering how he could express these depths and come out of a period of time so satisfied with himself. As he grew more able to rely on me to understand his efforts, the pet image died down. At the same time, his aggressions in the room, using me as one of the tools, increased.

Jake's play took on more and more feeling and intensity. My supervisor at the time had difficulty bearing witness to this work. At times during our weekly hour together, I was afraid that she might fall asleep from the toll that Jake's images put on her. One solution for me was to request the time at an all-clinic staff meeting to present Jake's material. Doing this gave me a small distance from which to listen to other clinical input. During this the time I also found a sandplay-based consultation group in the region.

Jake gets out the glass casket. He had identified the saber-tooth tiger as the Hunter. Two themes had organized themselves to make sense as one. The pet and the Hunter united as this new image, the one approaching the casket. This is a sign of organization occurring at the level of meaning.

"The saber-tooth tiger goes into the glass cage. The animals think he's dead. He's not. Not one of the animals knows what's in the box! (Jake lays an axe down near the cage.) They are making a war." *The parental war is now in image form, less worrisome but very agitating in this room. Jake has attempted to again lay the tension at the feet of those who need to resolve it. He has made a little headway.*

Containing the Transference

After this, Jake comes in full of energy. He cannot focus and demands that I check the clock for time and the window for his pick-up person. The room becomes tense. I feel as if every time a miniature moves about aggressively, my own body is dragged about and slams into other forces. I feel tired and am aware of being frustrated with Jake for something I cannot place. What is building, like being just outside the forces of a tornado? I watch these feelings, like speeding clouds, move me about. Looking back, the tension Jake brought in was his own crossroad: to stay put emotionally or to leap from his early perceptions into something not yet knowable.

Then Jake stops his play and looks directly at me. "Do you think my mom loves me?" Here is the heart of it, what the Hunter needed to find. When I try and send the question back to him, he shouts, "Do you think she does?" I respond, "It's hard, sometimes, to love. What do you know?"

"No." Jake pauses. "No. She doesn't love me. Sometimes, though, maybe she loves me." His aggression has shown a story origin, and as his truth surfaces, Jake falls into a depression. After this clear drop into his perceptions, Jake demands that I make a sign that this room is reserved only for him. Each session he adamantly locks it with a 3-inch skeleton key as he comes in, and unlocks it before we can leave. This locking and unlocking is a ritual that actively assists Jake's going deeper into the work he carries. Jake has sealed off the work now.

"Know what? I had the weirdest dream. I dreamed it was my birthday. And the animals had the weirdest dream. They dreamed they was alive." And so it seems—each week the animals do come alive.

Jake has entered a dreamtime of his own. The contractions and labor had brought both of us to this gate. Within our relationship, he will fully depend on his imagination to create that third space which is neither his reality nor his fantasy. This dream place dips from both and creates a reality that will carry him toward meaning that belongs utterly to him. As he goes more deeply into his hard work, the animals carry the array of mismatched feelings that often overwhelm Jake. This is where the repair of trust lies: in that original (again, primitive) place of where we begin. As newborns, "we" begin from an "us," which delivers us to a "me." Jake has found the "us," through his image of the Hunter, whose vital force

Jake: Building the Self

he has now embodied. He will need this strength to continue to the next dreamlike energies that might capture and bring his wholeness back to him. This innate ownership will be the treasure the Hunter is after. Again, this is Jake now relying on himself, *binding* to himself, because the witness is present. For the work to go where the child needs to be found, a witness is crucial. That throws us back into the definition of being *dependent*. To restate that meaning, to depend on: "to place trust or confidence [in]," "a subordination to something needed or greatly desired." The root meaning is "to hang from; to stretch."

During the next 3 months, Jake worked to find a way to recreate or produce images that might convey this self-recognition toward something tangible, something that carried the meanings he still pursued. I learned along beside Jake and did not always come upon what he was demanding in the moment. Our transference grew deeper, and I met with him twice a week to contain his neediness. His parents were fighting over him, over which house he would primarily live in. Jake's experience seemed to be ignored. In sitting with parents, I heard nothing that addressed Jake's own understanding of the divorce, or his needs. Jake played out his feelings of being invisible to this war going on over his head. But his heart was fully engaged.

Jake's urgencies, his needs to make use of me, and his overlapping and winding themes often disoriented my tracking. The unknowns remained constantly high and books were of no help in charting his course. I knew enough to remain in the work together. Still, I needed to know that I understood the meanings of the animals and the interactions between the miniatures, Jake and me. I made a long line, like a clothesline, on a sheet of paper, to which I continued to tape more paper as needed. Along this clothesline I wrote each session and its expressers: the bears, the dragons, the saber tooth. I drew colored lines from saber tooth to saber tooth, letting me know where that image surfaced and with whom. When Jake went to the dollhouse to formulate some perspectives he had on his family, they were pinned to the line, too. On this home-fashioned diagnostic clothesline, I also tracked his moods and sensations, using the spaces above and below the main line.

After placing a few month's worth of sessions and expressions on this clothesline, the themes became apparent. I continued on, realizing that this exercise as a new therapist was highly useful. I could nearly hear the wild animals and their voices speaking with the other crucial themes that interplayed. I could see when the saber tooth relented and stepped down, letting another voice address Jake's next leg of the journey. Without this effort, I am not sure I would have allowed Jake to go as deeply as he needed to: landing me the task of surrogate caregiver until he could finally rebuild the core human trust within that he was desperate to own. And when I say "allowed," I mean it. Children are not willing to go very far past the spaces where we, the witnesses, can accompany. It is in this sense that our own unconscious efforts, our fear of the unknown, and an overdependence on diagnostic tools can limit the work. And, although we cannot take it for granted, the child's intuitive awareness that stops him when no one else is coming along serves as a protection for the child.

The play turns to cutting up animals, dismembering them, saving heads. Jake wants me to take his key images, in the form of a miniature from one play or another, home with me. He brings a horse as a gift to me from home and compares it to a zebra that had early on tried to kick some walls down. Of this horse, Jake says, "There's big horses and small horses, like small kids." The horse dies because of the hard hooves of the zebra kicking him. The Hunter gets out tools and cuts the horse up. "They only want his feet, the powerful ones, and his head and his tail."

In some ancient rituals, the horse sacrifice was a fertility ritual. Keeping the head was intended for the most powerful. Jake

Jake: Building the Self

drops yet more deeply into his process. He cries when I will not take him to McDonald's. Then I am killed in the tray. Jake needs protection, and he is unsure that I can be that. He wants to drag me out into his external world, where protection is sorely lacking. We are at a crossroads of whether I am believable to his creation of self.

Jake goes on to play out his meaning of danger. When I tell him it is time to leave the room, he jumps into action, declaring, "I just have to put these pigs in yet. This mama pig is sad. She has just one baby (his younger sister?). This daddy pig has no babies. I say, 'Doesn't anyone want me?'"

He demanded that I rebalance when he begged me to go to McDonald's, when there was no amount of logic that would console him. I was ashamed of myself that I would not give in to this small request. At the same time, something in me felt so anxious that I knew it could not be the right thing. I did not know why, in the moment, but I knew I needed to hold on to this paradoxical battle in me. These moments of feeling lost and nonetheless having faith in the child's own urgent call to wholeness were my teaching spaces that gradually built my interior trust in each child's work.

During this developmental process, of recovering one's "primitive" origins, the play can vacillate from somewhat confrontive or disgusting play to positive metaphors of fairies and upbeat images. In Jake's work, play dynamics could change rapidly, leaving me confused and wanting to take over the driver's wheel on this out-of-control ride. Sometimes I felt whacked in my torso somewhere, only to be accused of "flying in space" and not fighting the good fight going on in the tray. I tried to keep up and simply to keep *in* his work, not worrying in the moment if I got what was happening so much as having faith that all of it meant something to Jake. Jake narrated the need to be united in our seeing into his process when he stated, *"I think you have my eyes, and I have your eyes. But my eyes are smaller."* Transference was heavy between us as we continued on, hunting for something that was gathering itself together even while we searched for it. A profoundly fragile balance rested uneasily between us: I was to be involved in his play while at the same time not actively engaged in the aliveness of the toys. The toys were alive by virtue of his own imagination. My job was to hold steady in trust and in resources of faith.

Alchemical Images

Now we enter the more ancient places of imagination. In Jungian and sandplay therapies this is called alchemy, which is very old in its symbolic meanings of transformation, and simultaneously means "a seemingly magical power or process of transmuting" (Edinger, 1985). "Alchemical images describe the process of depth psychotherapy, which is identical with what Jung calls individuation" (Edinger, 1985). Individuation is all about the task of becoming a "me." In that regard, alchemy provides us with a multilevel outline, an imaginal body into which we store our essential story of self.

In working with children, the toys "concretize" images into feeling states that the child might then throw our way. With enough trust the work is held while it builds a new requirement that, from inside the child, someone has *seen*. And Jake was in the grip of this individuation. At age 5, he needed to create the deep separateness that enables a child to begin the next big leap into social development. That step can be made in a healthy manner when the child has somewhat internalized the parent, who is still thoroughly available and standing by as the child grapples with the environments of school and friends. He would have to make of that process of self-discovery what he could on his own, since his parents were too engaged with their own life stressors to see his

Jake: Building the Self

highly sensitive needs. Jake would not make this step by himself. But he was risking the steps because of another's belief in him.

One reference identifies alchemy as "the symbolic process of turning a baser matter into gold; illumination or salvation." The meaning of alchemy and its parallel capacity to shed light on Jake's work is useful. Jake was indeed turning something base into gold, into his own empowerment. Looking upon Jake's intact images, he tackled his hunt for the gold, and then went on to create a personal relationship with a profoundly deep psyche that time will prove to be his greatest ally.

Jake has initiated images that confront his need of his own survival. At his level of work, survival is about one's felt truths being authentic and not able to be stolen by others. He now becomes the Dragon. He states, "<u>I'm</u> the dragon. I'm <u>it.</u>" When I naively ask if the dragon can hurt anyone, Jake states, "Well, I'm not playing yet. He didn't hurt <u>any</u>body. Now can I play?" (The gate into the playroom is locked. Now Jake will open his own trustworthy player within. I was premature.)

He identifies me as an Eastern goddess figure, whose name he says is "Smoke." He says he can pass through me and I remain and am not destroyed. "Everyone is afraid of me. I am strongest because I breathe fire." It seems as though I am to be the residue of this fiery image, someone who can be passed through and who has little say in the power of the creative fire itself. I have been given an appropriate role.

"Now you're turning into two things. You're the monster (still Smoke), and you're flying (the Eagle). I'm the dragon. And I'm Unicorn. You die. The eagle is buried." But, not all of me dies. *Jake is suddenly afraid. His aggression and its protections have personified, and those frightening feelings are him and me. They are no longer about us: they are us. He has buried some of me, and it takes a different kind of courage now for him to believe his untamed feelings will not somehow greatly harm me. This juncture* reveals how responsible I am for carrying Jake's wounded parts forward toward healing. At the same time, it is not about me, but rather about the space between us that Jake is currently fully relying on. As if he is a baby again, he hunts for my own ability to survive his destruction.

We have realized another marking stone on the pathway of his struggles: If he becomes separate, then what about Mom? Who will be there to assure her survival? I have come to find out in consult with Mom that she has been suicidal, and she wonders what effect that has had on her children. Jake has been fused with his mother's depressions, finding in himself too little strength to pull her to safety. This fused place, in separating from it, is worthy of his fear. But he pushes on.

Jake wants his mom to come, now. *He takes two dragons and moves us out of the room, to the porch. The container/room is too dynamic. I become the mom and the big dragon, and he is "Little Dragon." In order for him to blow fire I need to first blow fire into his mouth. Then Little Dragon practices, huffing and puffing, and after a bit he is able to blow fire. Jake also shyly has the little dragon nurse from the mama dragon.* Jake has attempted to oversee both his momma's presence and his own requirement of a "momma," a midwife, in this dream world he is utilizing. In following his needs to move his play to the porch (a transitional space), Jake does not collapse the dream he is creating. Instead, he is able to move that dream space forward, practicing to breathe the air in the deep transformative space between us.

Am I concerned during this time? Yes. I am alert, wary. I feel as though I am trespassing into a field not usually meant for me. I worry that I am providing some kind of ego-driven mothering. Looking back, I can see that I felt the edge of Jake's profound dependency on me. Inexperienced in being such a complete proxy for Jake's emotional mothering needs, I wonder if somehow I myself am making more of it than it is. My consultation support *group is just becoming trustworthy for me. The work feels so entirely mine, so unaided. I cannot afford to contain this alone, just in case I stumble. My consultation deepens as I demand more, since Jake needs the breathing in this space and we are so in sync that I cannot afford to slip too far and think my way into a separating dead end.*

The concerns I experienced, and was able to articulate in consultation, were voices of my own ego resistance. Our intellect may want to keep us in familiar landscapes safe from this burden of the child's feelings. We can look away from the child and still recognize the neighbor's house and the oak tree one block down. This is a more defined realness. To continue into the unknown, the ego must submit and rely on the trust in others, most of all, the child. In this, we are doing what we expect our clients to do: depend on an outside human being.

Jake had been projecting many unwanted parts and feelings into the toys in the room. Then slowly, as trust built in our relationship, he brought the work into active dynamics: Would I hold his anger? Would I be hurt when he killed me? Would he be strong enough to keep me at bay? In this hubbub of feeling states, Jake is thrown backward, so to speak, into the unattuned baby. With this openness in our relationship, we are mutually influenced as this dance, this effort, takes hold. It is as if by uncovering the communication of his behaviors, Jake is freed up to imagine himself again in the holding grasp of another, and in this grasp he is understood. Out of this trust coming from himself, he has a choice now to rebuild, and to construct in the remodel what had been missing.

In this developmental individuation, Jake has slain the wounding mother in order to create and then express, out from this imaginal space between us, an internalized caring mother. By "slaying," I mean that he has faced his awful fears that he is capable of hurting an essential person with his hateful feelings.

To be clear, this internal caring one is not me. I am the proxy, the other in the dance, while Jake subsumes a deep protection from his dreaming self. This effort is both introjective and regressive. Introjection is "the process of incorporating characteristics of a person into one's own psyche unconsciously" (American Heritage Dictionary, 1992).

Regression occurs as a kind of setback that is caused by depression or submission to something in the present. The present links us to the past harm, and we re-enter that past to unlatch ourselves from harm done. Our visit to this past can reorganize what had taken us away from our own primal selves. Regression is in essence a stepping back in order to leap forward, such as is done in pole vaulting. Jake is now using both of these dynamics. In his imagination, I am the midwife/mother that brings a new kind of nourishment to this "baby dragon." Jake had projected his aggressions onto animal after animal, and death and burial had been dominant. He had landed in the original space, the primitive and chief place, where dependency had not been present enough. Jake's false bravado was waning as he faced such core needs. He is molting. Molting is a most vulnerable transition between an old shell covering and no new shell yet present.

Parent Consultations

His mother was struggling in her own identity crisis that drew her attention away from Jake, during a self-identifying time in his growth. Jake was in the developmental process that would focus on building his own individuality. At one point, when Jake's depression was at its deepest, I struggled with my ongoing anger toward his parents. Later on I would understand that I was feeling the feelings of Jake's own desperate needs to be seen. At the time, however, I could hardly tolerate the monthly consultations I held with them. Jake's need to be witnessed in his perceptions of being the family pet were in me, too. As he tossed and turned between depression and rage, so did I. I knew enough to understand that I was containing the "us" between Jake and me. The mutual field of mistrust in his parents revealed itself in parent consultations as a kind of loss of thought, an inability to form thoughts into words. My own seeming loss of intelligence was confusing to me, and it made me less and less willing to sit with them. I blamed them for Jake's loss of calm self and wanted to tell them I would yell and kick too for the poor attention he was receiving. I had to hold back feelings that might be haphazardly concealed as education in dealing with his tantrums. Jake himself was letting me know he did not feel heard. Sitting with his parents, I did not feel heard, either. I am not sure now whether I was or not, since my anger with these two adults was so present.

The dynamic of parent/infant identification is a bass note played in infant attachment, and when that base is missing, the song that is played is missing its harmony. Schore addresses this dynamic in his work with attachment, calling this dyad, with their "spontaneous gestures," a mark of securely attached babies. Spontaneity carries that rhythm that we addressed earlier, the resonance that flows between the mother/infant duo. Schore harkens back to Winnicott, and he quotes Winnicott saying the attuned mothers are "giving back to the baby the baby's own self" (Schore, 2003).

This is the best art of play therapy: to "give back to the child the child's own self." When we refresh some worn out words, we are able to see more closely how hard repair work is for a child. And regression as used here is the return to a more primitive structure, that is, the relational dyad of the infant-mother: to begin again, and along the way to make repair. What makes this period so primitive is that in the child's first attachments, to which Jake and I had returned, there is no filter but the otherness of the mother. There is no other that takes the overwhelm, detoxifies it, and returns it to the baby's felt self in a digestible manner. That filtering system is the well-being of the baby, and without it, a myth begins that can go as deep as feeling unloved.

Even earlier, prior to this imaginal work in which Jake was engaged, he had projected his frightening uncertainties about being a loveable person via his aggressive behaviors. He counted on someone slowing down this form of communication, his bodily aggression, to find out what he was really saying. In this, it is fair to say that Jake had been projecting his fears outward, onto his family members, to let them know how afraid he was.

I felt the integrity of where we were going together. There is so much room for enactment here: simply giving in to the ride of being so profoundly connected with a child or keeping too much distance so that the child feels unattended. In hindsight, I can see that Jake and I entered this when he demanded that he take home the saber-tooth tiger. I said I would bring a box that was special to me, and that he, the saber tooth, would stay there whenever Jake chose. I told Jake that I would also bring something of mine to keep in this box. This is when Jake began locking the door with that enormous key, naming what and why he needed to do so. After this initial ritual, he would take the wooden box down and place it abutting the tray. He checked to see the contained objects and quietly held them for a tiny bit. My notes say that it seemed he was weighing them, noting their realness. Then he would begin to play. I understood that Jake had accepted the containment and the no-McDonald's voice, and that his wailing to go out into the community had been addressed. In this, I had passed a profound transference test, of holding firm to the container that was myself. That boundary was a mutual agreement that rested between us now and manifested in an imaginally locked door. Both of us slipped more deeply into Jake's work. This is what I refer to as the integrity of the work. The wooden box holding us together was the ritual that spoke to the fidelity between us. A kind of faith in the process itself entered the work. Jake's mom said he had quite suddenly stopped throwing tantrums and demanding impossible things, and she was delighted and puzzled.

Today Jake states he has two problems. He describes them. He puts a fence through the tray. "This fence is real, more real than you. Smoke can be bad. She can just rise up, phew-phew, in smoke." *Jake goes on to describe that his older sister plays tricks on him, making him hunt for his dad when his dad is gone. I think out loud, that not only are tricks being played, but in fact, Dad must be gone again. Jake goes quiet.* "Yep."

Phew-phew. Gone again.

After playing out more empowerment, Jake reenters his journey. He draws a dragon on paper. "His name is Red-Eye because he has a red eye. Where did he get it from? God just made him that way. Cuz God just had to make a red eye." *He asks me,* "What would you say to the dragon? You're calling for help."

I respond, "I would say, 'I'm brave. I have a kind heart.'"

Jake: "You wouldn't say that! You'd say Yikes! And you'd just run. You'd be sooo scared!"

Me: "You're right, Jake. I <u>would</u> be scared."

"Yeah, cuz this dragon is so powerful. He's mad. If you were in the castle, would you not be scared?"

Me: "Only if I had some magic, then I wouldn't be scared."

Jake: "Yeah, your ghost magic. He'd rip at you and then you'd pass through." *Jake's tantrums and aggressions are being defused.*

Jake had taped a large dinosaur down onto paper, to keep it from kicking anyone. He identifies this: "That means BIG Work." *Then he continues on with his drawings.* "Know who I am? The dragon. Who's the snake? You. You get too close to the dragon. The dragon blows fire and burns off his head." *I am the headless one now, unable to think any way out of this. Will I survive at the mercy of this power? The page fills up with redness, while*

Jake excitedly tells me, "The dragon can do this! I didn't think he could, but he could*! He has smoke coming out of his nose, too. They thought he was sick. But he's not. All this fire barely hits the sun, out and out." As Smoke, Jake has taken me on, breathing me out without any illness. All that rests in our relationship is becoming tolerable to Jake, even though Jake was not sure this could happen.*

That baby dragon that practiced on the porch has mastered his greatest asset, of fire-breathing, of creating change. Can you imagine how alive this dragon is? Dragons are so powerful. So much so that Jake himself is taken off guard by what the dragon is capable of. This is where we land together, the child and the therapist, in a world full of surprise, risking wonderment together over the power of the designated driver of the moment. Jake's description of this is perfect:

"My brain is up here (points to his head) and it stays up here and my heart is in here (points to his chest), but sometimes it can go up to my brain and talk."

Another session: "This dragon is awesome! Very red! You're the prince. You're in the tall tower. I'm burning you. You jump into the water. A king fish saves you. But then he eats you up."

"I'm blowing more and more fire. The castle is all red. Now the king fish is burned, even though he was in the highest tower. You're in the castle and you'll never get out. Oil spilt out of the sky. It hit me! Oil is burning my leg!–Magic comes from the castle. The dragon wants bad magic, and the castle wants good magic. The dragon is dying. Do you want me to die? You're dead already in the castle. Do you?" I say no.

The Fisher King Legend

On this day, Jake's images allude to the Fisher King, who was also struck in the thigh and wounded. This Fisher King is the king

Jake: Building the Self

of the Holy Grail legend. The hunt for the Holy Grail is a myth of the great Quest, ultimately for the psyche or soul. The legend has many religious and spiritual meanings. While it is too much of a stretch to say Jake knew anything about the Grail in his five-year-old self, his unconscious had tapped into a universal myth that held him in its intentions of the Knight hunting for the Right Question. This is one of the deepest and most creative uses of the imagination. As with dreams, we tap into a larger myth that embraces all of us universally. This universality is available and useable by any one of us when needed.

A month later, Jake states that he needs to draw treasure. He has survived the violence of his own power, that of fire, as have I. Treasure signifies a turn in the work, although Jake is not done with the forces of being the dragon. Nor is he done with the gold. He continues:

"Where's gold? I'm the dragon, drawing the gold. Eyes got to be red, and also his tail." Jake is the dragon, and the dragon is the creator. Jake instructs me to write, "The cobra snake and the dragon were fighting over a treasure. The dragon blew open the lock with his fire."

"You know what came out of the treasure? Oil. It killed the dragon. It burned up the snake too." Jake draws the sun. "Boom! It accidently hit the sun. You know what happened? Red stuff came out. (This and the dragon's red eye are the same.)" This is too "hot" for Jake. In baby talk, he creates a hero, which calms him. What is this red? The blood in the body? Fire? Certainly, we are in the center of an embodying process, of a little boy who goes back and regathers all of himself in order to claim the gold of his life. All this redness and its creator, the sun, is the greatest of fire. It is the alchemical power that turns metal into gold. It demands heroism and boldness.

Oil. In alchemy and in ancient rituals, oil was used in "consecration, and a preservation against corruption; for high

223

priests, kings, etc.; the grace of God; balm" (de Vries, 1984). Jake knew none of this taproot of the image that he chose. However, he continued to tap into that deeper human myth, which Jung called the collective unconscious. Jake's images seemed to need this force to back him up as he struggled in the container where he had locked both of us. What Jake did know was that oil is a substance that can even overcome the dragon. Jake will continue to make use of this ingredient as he moves deeper and deeper into his origin story. The dragon, Jake, has committed to a force that would oversee his aggressions while taming his infant omnipotence.

Jake spent several months practicing this new self-understanding. At times he was full of aggression, while at other times he worried that his being angry hurt his mom right in that moment of his play. His efforts to be neither a good nor a bad part worked at him. His calmer behaviors held in his home. The "violence" had a place in which to be understood. The inner war was forging a new entity, a child who might believe in his worth.

At one point he puts a chalice in the tray and fills it with sand. This, he tells me, is "salt for the dragon. It makes him have fire."

Salt has been discussed from many angles in Jung's books. Salt often serves as a centering symbol of transformation.

Jake's difficulty had been located in his comprehension, whether real to others or not, that he was unloved. It has taken a tremendous powering up for Jake to face this internal destructive reality. And the salt he places in the chalice is the vortex of alchemical, transformational change.

There is an immense number of references to alchemical processes in Jake's work. It is not my goal to identify most of those. What is intended here is that we witness Jake's journeying ensconced in an inner world of imagination. He connects to an unconscious and powerful struggle to separate from his belief that he is unloved and unlovable. Achieving this, he treks on to gain access to a connection with some part in him that knows who he is. And activating this wisdom enables Jake to tolerate and then redeem his own self-trust and self-love.

Near the end of this round of his therapy, Jakes speaks of being all the animals, both good and bad. He says this is hard. He fills a fridge with salt. I ask what it is about salt that they need. His reply: "Salt is the most magic! It makes things happen. This room has lots of salt in it."

"Salt is the secret of the work... the substance in which matter and spirit seemed to come together. Salt as center is most significant" (Raff, 2000). Alchemy states that "the salt of the earth is the soul." Jung, in the *Mysterium Coniunctionis*, states, "Just as the world-soul pervades all things, so does salt. It fulfills the main requirement of an arcane substance, that it can be found everywhere. It represents the feminine principle of Eros, which brings everything into relationship" (Jung, 1970).

Jake's "salt" is in the fridge, which opens when we are hungry. His resources are kept fresh and available. Jake can now concretely speak of his reality. He has developed a strong enough ego to speak *from*. He says he feels frustrated.

"I can talk some about frustration, but let's leave this room first. My dad tells me too much. He tells me how he hates Mom's boyfriend and how he hates not living with her. It's too much. He says, 'It's your problem too.' But I say 'NOT'—not out loud, but in here, in my imagination. I say inside, it's not my problem. Mom, though, talks a lot, too. She tells me about Dad, about her needing to live alone. I have problems out there, lots of problems. Things aren't right. I don't have problems here, except I like to put things away right. That's all. But I don't have the other problems here."

After more practicing within the containment of our relationship, Jake plays a game he had played many times. He always had asked me what would happen next, and when I would not say, he got quite upset with me. At one point in the work, he had celebrated that of course I did not know what would happen.

In his closing moments, he asks me again what animal or car or ship is him. I respond with a contented "Jake, I don't know!" To which he states, "What! You always know!" But now, Jake caringly gives me clues so that I can *find out* from his wisdom, what is right, and who is him. With his help, I can understand Jake, while holding my position outside of him. My care has a "good enough" magic now, but is not stronger than his own. He has reclaimed the ability to love himself.

And to this end, Jake creates a picture of a butterfly. Then he uses the elemental colors of lava—red, smoke-gray, oil-black, and yellow-gold—on a separate paper. Over all of these he creates a rosebush. The rose is one of the universal symbols of the Self. Jake dots his creation with reds. "This is my rose-berry bush. It's growing." The dragon's red eye had found a way to create more of living. Jake had won a very deep battle.

Learning From the Child's Self

Jake was one of my deep, early teachers. His frank confrontations, such as "I'm not playing yet…" or "Do *you* know what happens next?!" gave me the markers of patience and listening an extra heartbeat or two past what I had heard. His excitement as he grew to trust me inside his work brought satisfaction to both of us. These moments of feeling lost and nonetheless having faith in the child's own urgent call to wholeness were my teaching spaces that gradually built my interior trust in each child's work.

I played such a surrogate during those many months that I had to tighten up my watch for both of us. My more advanced consultation group was an additional support. I knew I was crisscrossing the "usness" of him and me, back and forth, weaving together a crosshatch that would become a protective barrier for him. But while we did this work, I was the boundary, the fence line that kept his younger fragments from overwhelming him emotionally. This was Jake's own tray image of the fence that was "real, more real than you." Jake would gradually own this boundary as his own, and as a creation from within him. Every session he faced the hard work of rebuilding his trust in another so that he could internalize an image of wholeness. It seemed as though nothing escaped his nervous regard. He was always correcting me, sharply demanding of me, reminding me to "be here now." I felt my own nervous regard, my feelings of ineptness, and my own questions about where he and I were going in this work together. I would step back to see, only to be snapped back into its demands, and knowing far less than I thought I should know. Jake's work urged me to provide the both of us with a map into the interior.

Jake entered his healing work with a fierceness that put me inside his fire, both emotionally and symbolically. I felt that he was drawing his strength to do this leg of the journey from my very bones. When Jake locked the playroom door with that large ancient-looking key, I felt the "we are in and everyone else is out" requirement in my own breathing. I was not sure I knew what to do with such a complete separation from others. My body felt the pull of entering a solo run with this little boy, and there were no words to let me know where we might land. Over and over, Jake's hard work took me away from knowing, and dropped me into a bigger domain, of faith in relationship.

I know that Jake grew up with difficulties: his "problems" were not resolved. His parents went though many moltings, and Jake seemed to remain intensely close to their feeling states. What he had tried to throw out of himself, in kicking and tantrums and aggression, were the ingredients of his own acute sensitivities that had overwhelmed him. And these were the elements that sent him in search of his own holy grail: Am I loved.

We needed to go about grieving that he could never save either of his parents from themselves. He could, however, build the stamina from his own inside-to-outside, that would house his sophisticated capacity for empathy. I had the luxury of checking in with Jake another two times prior to his tenth birthday, when his environments intruded too far into his status as a child. As an adult, Jake is successfully married and carrying on a life far away from his family of origin.

CHAPTER 12

Ruthie: Challenges Between Us in Co-transference

At age 9, Ruthie had had to undergo surgery in her brain for a tumor. Although she had been very active in sports and outdoor hiking, these interests had been stopped. Ruthie came to see me because of depression which, in such a young child, was disturbing to her parents.

She begins her work quietly, seeming not to have a lot of connection to her work, or to me. We often sit together quietly while she steadily works in the tray. At some point, Ruthie begins a series of trays that work with the skeletons. Later on, she lays the axe down by the skeleton. I wonder if we are in the body's domain of experience, in the body's betrayal of what had been innocent safety. Something had invaded. The axe may be the venue of entry to find her meaning of this invasion.

Ruthie is narrating her story more and more. As she does this, she counts on my presence more. She is willing to use me as a witness, and at times the toys address an overwhelming fear that remains from her journey. The skeletons and death figures become spiders and other insects, perhaps those who are creepy-crawly feelings.

In the heart of her work, Ruthie selects a Buddha figure with an incense bowl. She chooses carefully and has a detailed cast of figures. I sense a growing tension from Ruthie. Her continuous glances in my direction let me know that my attention must be sure-footed. I align with something more tense and apprehensive coming toward us. There are snakes, a first-aid kit, weapons, bridges. As she puts in a temple gateway, she states, "If you go around this, it's bad luck. You have to go through it."

"The god is being shot. Gods of the forest who come out of your nature come out now. You have angered the gods!" Ruthie shouts. An axe hurls through the air. A man who has attempted to cross the bridge is cut through with two stakes (perhaps the two surgeries Ruthie had faced). Ruthie steps over to where I am sitting to be sure that, from my angle, it is clear that the stakes have hit the head and neck of this man and that I clearly see that. Then Ruthie takes the axe and, glancing directly at me, has it cut into the man's head. The man says, "I'm taking someone with me!"

At this point, I hear my own neck pop. I am suddenly in deep pain, where my birth trauma lives. Ruthie has clearly done a perfect job in demanding that I share in her experience. She finally has someone to take with her. I silently weigh in on Ruthie's voice, her demand to take someone with her, and my sudden clash of pain. I recognize that I now share in her pain, body to body.

The spiders now become very active. Eventually Ruthie builds a sort of map. It is a round container drawn in the sand, with several compartments. She carefully places a spider in one major area and the Buddha from the previous work in another. There is also a treasure chest, and some trophy awards. To me this feels like a diagram of Ruthie's brain, both containing the scary things and honoring the gods who had been angered.

How do we learn from children what it is that is needed? How do we best use the skills and tools for which we rummaged about in graduate programs, workshops, consultations, and life in general? What is it to this tracking of images and symbols that builds upon itself, over and over, so that in the tracking we come to understand themes and processes that reveal the nature of each child's internal world?

Dynamics in the Co-transference

Transference, working in a shared field of energy, is at—or within—the heart of relatedness. In Latin, the two roots of –fer- in transference, and –re- in relating, point to a single verb meaning "to carry, bear, bring, support, endure" (American Heritage Dictionary, 1992). The notions of relating and relatedness assign one meaning as "having a close harmonic connection" (American Heritage Dictionary, 1992). As we shuffle these implications into a path we might follow, we find ourselves heading straight into the heart of what matters most: relationship. Transference exacts of us that as we head into—or land in—the shared feelings with another, we need to have built at least some understanding of its activities and its intense mutual feeling states. In transference, we are both bearing and being borne along mutually shared, implicit meanings. We are together, harmonious more in the sense of resounding together, back and forth, than merely in being pleasingly harmonious. Harmony in this instance can mean a struggle, a burden being lifted that has been very painful and now has two to carry it. And in that two-ness, the child really knows that we are an authentic other that is sharing the load, being receptive to that which we are given to comprehend. Relationship conveys a mutuality, a shared burden, so that when two reach into what requires attending, something new approaches. Remember early on where attachment also came from root words of stretching and reaching out. Relationship might appear to be another noun. But in the space it holds, between you and me, it dances.

Ruthie has found her own wound: losing innocence to an illness that stole her sense of unconditional protection. Her own depression had worked on this betrayal. But the meanings kept being too big, too abstract, for Ruthie to comprehend. Her play and its images bring her in connection with what it is she needs to express. Her communication is so thorough that we bear it together now.

We are trusted to remain in this receptive state until the child lets go of, exhales, the solitary struggle that had taken hold and separated the child from himself. Transference has mysterious elements within it, because by its very nature, we partially let go of the bounded shape of ourselves. My neck popping with the weight of Ruthie's effort became the visceral overlap. This connection is a being, not a doing, and it becomes difficult to pin down. It moves about with two people attending to it and is not primarily under the government of the therapist's left-brain approaches. When we think about bearing something, it works two ways. First, can we bear feelings and bodily responses that seem foreign to us? And can we bear the burden of the child's troubled heart long enough for something that we do not yet know to realize itself? We relax into a receptive state that trusts the child's own inner world with its news from the interior (Bollas, 1987). And that news will surface because we are there waiting, holding forth that trust. It is as if we have arrived in the child's own interior, and having gotten ourselves there, there is little to do but *be,* which is a very active state of being. In this state, we are made use of. We are animated by the child's own wisdom, a knowing that is deeper by far than daily events and relationships. This inclusion of ourselves in the child's world gives the child someone to speak with in images, metaphor, or words, from the profound yearnings and cares of being human. And in this space the child remembers his own wholeness, his own capacity to trust himself.

Looking back now, I might articulate something of what happened when Ruthie's pain entered my body. She and I had developed a relationship of trust and integrity. Ruthie relied on the toys to speak in her behalf. On the day when Ruthie set up the portal from which those gods would visit, her images had established full-on acceptance that the toys would be the representatives to her announcement. *"You have to go **through** the temple's gateway"* revealed who was really coming. Ruthie continued to glance at me, as if to say, *"Are you still with me? Can you come along?"*

As she found me still present, she ignited the space with her call: *"I'm taking someone with me!"* The toys would hold the presence of some mutual field that thoroughly included me. I took in the pain so much so that my body was included. This inclusion is what Ruthie required in order to be found.

The challenge here is that as we touch upon the real, interior dance of transference; we can no longer speak about functionality and procedure. In the transference that visits between therapist and child, we no longer assume that we will understand the details of what healing reveals. We count on faith, on waiting and holding open a space that accepts information that we ourselves had not thought. This faith has not entered the behavioral blessings of a treatment plan. Instead of words, this world creates a shared-mindedness from the implicit, less-than-verbal realms of the two of us. The child is still so close to his nonverbal state of being, that primitive world of the body, imagination, and spontaneity as one creative blend. As we approach this creativity, the degree of trust that has been established will be the key that allows us in. And located in this trust is the understanding that I have not come to change you. You have taken a chance with me so that you might change you.

We are the dependable presence. In the original states of a child's full dependency, what was lost in trauma is the trust and faith that someone has been there, calling a name that registers as "me," this "I" who is being known. When no one is there, trust is overcome by fear. Fear removes the child from ownership of her perceptions. Lacking ownership, she becomes lost. Being lost a long time creates chronic trauma, a perceived "me" without the faith that you will find this "me." Being remembered, having implicit, unthought memory that stores another's love of us, travels this deep. Being remembered is absolutely dependent on relationship, and the meanings we give to memory exist out of the underlying forces of relationship. Relatedness is all of this: being known, being loved, and the receptivity of another that acknowledges that we are real. And in this relatedness, we become able to be real to ourselves.

The Therapist's Self Work

Transference requires first and foremost the presence of a structure within the therapist. That structure will be our own inner guidance, the map of self, as we utilize our awareness of injuries on behalf of another. The structure we will need is from having done and from continuing to do our own work. Working away at what drivers propel us about in the unconscious, we learn about who we ourselves were as children. Recognition of this brings about awareness and receptivity that we still carry the map of that child somewhere inside. The essence of a "me" does not significantly shift over a lifetime. I know, for example, that as an adult Jake remained true to his unusual capacity to intuit others' feelings and needs. He had a number of childhood occasions that pushed hard on his innate gifts. He rose to those challenges.

As we bring compassion to the selves we accommodate, we increase compassion for these aspects of ourselves. This empathy will become available to others as we comprehend our own injuries. Comprehension and empathy for where we have been walking builds an increasing sense of order. We can offer sympathy and compassion to our own foibles and clumsy steps. This empathy builds a more unified sense of self from the inside out. An internal structure sustains our own trust in the processes of others because we have learned to trust our own thoughts, feelings and perceptions more of the time. We become more capable of offering our compassion without collisions between two worlds of unconsciousness.

The structure we build in the co-transference includes an ability to observe ourselves with a bit of neutrality and some good amount of empathy. It is as if when the child demands that we "get" that child's experiences in the home, we become of two minds. One mind is our own, observing that we are feeling clumsy or confused or not ourselves. This mind needs empathy for ourselves. The other mind, while also our own, houses the child's own experiences. We feel feelings that are less definable, shaky, possibly critical of the child and/or ourselves. This two-mindedness needs our own ability to observe itself in this quandary at least a little. It also needs a supervisor or consultant who perceives that we are struggling to hold this duality as a single-minded therapist. That outside entity needs to have empathy for our predicament in order for us to be safe to explore it and find ourselves in this twofold space. I cannot emphasize enough the importance of an experienced supervisor. If our own supports withdraw during this time in the child's work, we will likely experience the child's own helplessness and confusion more profoundly. We will perhaps need to withdraw from some or all of the containment of the child's own work.

Our own support is that important. It can put the work we are witnessing at risk. To be clear, part of our own internal structure includes the trust we have placed in our professional witnesses. Having a person who keeps our trust in the process intact allows us to be more fully present as we respond to the demands of the child's lost self coming into view. The structure here points to the therapist's own capacity to maintain an inner space for the child's material. Structure implies the therapist's ability to contain load-bearing information from the child. The information given replicates the child's own experiences and meanings of those experiences, into the comprehension of the therapist.

There are risks, sometimes more and other times less, in the shared space of co-transference. One danger is that when our own hurts are triggered, our work can enter the shared space without our awareness. This causes outbreaks, potentially toxic times when work is not getting done. Instead, the child may feel a familiar need to take care of our intrusiveness, just as he has done with his intimate caregivers. The boundaries that might lead to empowerment are flooded, and the child receives an unstable therapist. In the periods where the child has risked vulnerability in order to make a second attempt at being seen, what is being reinforced is the core nature of the wound: that of not being known or understood as separate and whole. Having no guide who steadily keeps to the child's course and urgencies may well bring about failure. In supervising master-level interns, this is a radar signal that is always on, since working in image and metaphor can more naturally bring on the child's desire to reveal his truths. In itself, flooding the shared space with one's own reactions is not necessarily a failure. These are the risks we must take in order to reveal and come to know this landscape of mutual space. How can we learn of our own limitations unless we experience them with the very children we hope to serve? The real failure is in not seeing this understanding or seeing it and not immediately correcting it.

If these core realities are not in place, particularly in working with children, it becomes wisest to stay in the domain of attachment and behavioral shifts that do not easily encourage co-transference (although it is by no means protection against its occurrence). We may cause further harm when we fail to maintain our own struggles of awareness. This may sound harsh, but we are at all times charged with the task of the child's physical, emotional and psychic safety.

Requirement of Faith in the Child's Self

We want to know about the child's faith in us that is and is not about our own beliefs. Undefended expectations that we will truly grasp the child's needs and meanings approach us from the child's interior world, and ask us to remain available to its depth. If we go spiraling out into ungrounded views of alchemical realities (which can be important, but is no place in which to place our overwhelms), we have escaped the child's own presence. What we experience truly *is* the child's own faith in the child's self, and it will speak in symbols that need us to listen with some understanding rather than adoration.

In the mirroring that requires such full attunement, we are the assisting individuals who are called upon to mend the preverbal wounds in the child. Being nonverbal, these wounds carry a power that is primal in their yearning to be known by another. Remember the requirement of the infant's mother, to respond to the baby's implicit experiences with her own attuned mirror. She responds with just enough difference that the baby has a little room in which to develop a separate self. Just a little. She absorbs her baby's communications, refreshes them, and offers them back in palatable form as she responds. This is the rhythm of "yes, and" I accept you and your needs, and I am a self that sends your you-ness back to you. This is also the therapeutic transference: we accept the perceptions and feeling states of the child, shift the load a little bit, and return that labor to its owner in a more digestible form. We are not the owner. We are, at times and momentarily, the stand-ins within the child's implicit experiences. Our small amount of difference is the energy that sustains the growing symbolic activities that will in time, create and organize the child's own healing and the child's ownership of his process.

Implicit Memories Alive in the Present

The memories of the past are still alive and acting as the behaviors we see. Though there might not be words attached to the memories, the meanings are what need expression, and one way or another, those meanings are expressed. The child's behaviors are the visibility of her needs, where the past remains unresolved and in need of insight. Play and relationship pull away at the experiences that are attempting to remain past, but which continuously appear in the present, hungering for comprehension. The child carries that insight, but little will come of it unless a safe relationship carries the responsibility of what the child feels and knows instinctively. This is not to be confused with cognitive awareness. When we confuse instinctive knowledge with conscious awareness, we will make demands on the children to explain themselves, not express themselves. In demanding that the child act responsibly, we use name-calling like "She is just being manipulative" or "He always does this when he does not get his way." We cease to be patient with the part that is our own job: that of listening and then connecting the dots for an image that is to be tested by the child for its clarity. Behaviors will not be pacified until they feel understood. The therapist is the negotiator, able to listen and attend to the unspoken language that goes on behind the behavior. The therapist represents the child's intentions to the home and school environments, having heard from the child what hurts.

Voices From the Unconscious

Here is the crux of transference and imagination: the past remains unconscious, except in its urgent expression, until the relationship that was meant to be in that past experience becomes available now. A little 4-year-old boy that I worked with long ago, Justin, had witnessed an inordinate amount of physical abuse. His neurological systems were constantly overwhelmed. The preschool called me and asked if I could observe this child's responses to noise. As I arrived, Justin was tearing down the hallway, pulling down a large cabinet as he ran past me. The staff was chasing him in an attempt to stop further chaos. I told them to stop in their tracks. It seemed that everyone's brains were unable to think. After telling the teachers to secure the outside in case Justin ran out, I asked for a blanket and followed Justin into a room at the end of the hallway. As I entered, he prepared to run again. In a low voice, I told Justin I would not follow where he went, but I would make sure he stayed safe. I laid down the blanket and said he must be really really scared. The blanket might help him get comfortable. Then I backed out of the room, to the doorway. Justin watched me, a frightened little animal in a corner. I understood that the staff wanted so badly to comfort him, but his survival brain was on fire.

I started working with Justin in the playroom. His alertness to my movement helped me to experience how profoundly frightened he had been. We gradually worked on having his arms and legs talk to me about being scared, and when they were scared, they ran, kicked, and grabbed things. Slowly Justin somehow understood that his arms and legs knew a lot about his fears. Between sandtray image-building, I asked him what he had heard that week from his body. He and I had our bodies talk together, an arm to an arm. The sadness I felt was deep. My body seemed to "get" his body's information. Near the end of our work, Justin told me, "My legs aren't scared anymore." I asked him how he knew that. "Cuz they walk. They don't kick. They like me." What a handful for a child, now 5, to grasp, and then to allow someone else to take in the cornered self this little body had experienced. Now it seemed Justin moved about in physical space with more confidence, which spoke to others through a sharp decrease in aggression. Through a relationship that slowed down and steadied itself in the language Justin had learned to use for safety, Justin found access to the origins of a self prior to being in constant alarm.

It is the relationship that upends implicit memory, as the therapist takes on the identified other in the dance that was meant to be before. It can happen in the here and now, and in its occurrence, the child updates meaning, embedding this new allowance of the self as being what was needed all along. This is difficult to get words around, as it becomes a paradox, necessarily, of both past and present: old map of relationship and new map of relationship, all crowding in at the same place and time. And this is right where it must sit for a spell as the child absorbs a new realization: I am ok! I am loveable because you love me!

Limitations of Play Therapy

True play exists between two people. Old meanings slip out, into the toys, right here and right now, between us. The toys are now capable of becoming symbols, lit up with the tasks they are assigned by the interior of the child's needs. I am a required part of the equation. Not just any "I." This "I" must have the skills that foster awareness and the heart to risk being changed by the creative efforts of a child. The transference will then have worked its profound shifts.

At times it is crucial to identify the boundaries children bring to the work. It is clearly not an option to go into image-work with all children. Again, a child taught me about this. Jon was 7, and his behaviors were unpredictable. He moved from laughter to tears quickly. School staff could not understand his needs, and his mom was not able to say what caused these mood swings. I began his work in the sandtray room, which was typical. I noted that his mother had been drinking heavily for his first 4 years of life, and I credited his behaviors as a need to find new landing places with her, deeper attachment, and repair. I needed to get information on a fetal alcohol syndrome diagnosis also, although Mom said she did not drink during this pregnancy.

Jon began to disintegrate further in the use of miniatures and sand. He wanted to turn off all the lights and work with a flashlight, which caused him to nearly panic. My own gauge inside was sending alarms more often. We went outside the building, in part for me to see if natural environments would soothe this growing imbalance. Jon began talking with the worms, urging them to find their moms. Of course this could support my theory of diagnosis. But now both of us were getting lost, unhinging. I required his family to get him into a children's facility. Jon required 2 weeks of in-hospital care and daily cognitive mapping while the medical crew fashioned medications that stabilized him. In the process of this learning curve, illusions of grandeur disappeared. Jon taught me that I am one on a significant bell curve of child professionals who often do their best work as individuals in a team.

I supported Jon's parent through the many changes that were required, being a backdrop to the team she needed to build for her son. That support was highly useful to the family construct. My style of therapy, the room as container, and what I had to relationally offer to Jon were not compatible. My trust in my own capacity to guide Jon to safe ground was not taking hold. There was little to no grip between us, and as I slid with him, I realized that the image-ridden environment I was offering was only loosening up a fragile hold he had on his internal reality. Jon seemed to long for me to "catch" him, while at the same time his emotions were becoming less and less real to himself. His monologue with the family of worms was heartbreaking, but we could not make any use of his efforts. There was nothing that allowed an entry. The more I attempted, it seemed the more frightening I became to him. I needed to make a thorough, clear decision to find psychiatric care. Even though there are many times that a good therapist can shoulder the family system thoroughly enough to pull that system to firmer ground in this model, this was not one of those. Jon would need more cognitive approaches, to help him learn intervention skills for his own jumpy brain.

The decisions we must make in our work with young children are often this elusive and demanding. Children will grab a hand that seems safe and head on out, even in the most strenuous of circumstances. There are no firm guidelines in this question of who we serve. Experience and a good consult team may be our best allies. I will not hesitate to work with a child whose family is also willing to work, even when that child may suffer from her own disabilities. A team for the family might need to be built. Developmental education might be highly useful. There are many layers that a good therapist can offer to walk with the child toward increased health. As a team gathers together, I will be more able to see if my own models will help this child, or if I have been the bridge that has strengthened the parents in finding the right fit.

Working with Children Born Addicted

Another of my great teachers was a little girl who had been born addicted. After going through her own withdrawal, she proceeded to lose her parents to their continuing addictive choices. Four-year-old Mylah had layers of trouble: loss, a compromised neurology, and her own physical and emotional meaning of environmental failures. She had spent weeks in a newborn intensive care unit (NICU) in a darkened room where caregivers urged her to eat. Because of her experiences of newborn addiction, Mylah had complex failure to thrive. Those brain signals were turned off. One reason I chose to work with her was clear to me. Her adoptive parents were on board with her interior challenges, to the best of their ability. They needed someone to see into their family system and to understand the array of confusion that Mylah brought with her. They wanted to know how far they could reach and what tools were needed in creating changes that supported this little one. So we began our journey. Adopted mom sat just outside the playroom, ready to take hold of Mylah should she take off, and simultaneously ready to give her a hug every 10 minutes or so. Her presence kept Mylah facing the relationship between the two of us. My first focus was to see if we could emphasize attachment. If we could accomplish something there, Mylah might have more solid grounding in the other arenas in her life.

She and I spent inordinate amounts of time fixing meals, stirring things together, dishing them up on plates, and pretending to eat them. Chairs placed around the play table seated baby dolls, and they seemed to argue for enough food. We often sent out a full plate for Mom, too, which accomplished some sharing and more importantly, a check as to mom's continued presence. I attended as the number of babies increased, their needs becoming more and

Ruthie: Challenges Between Us in Co-transference

more pronounced, their efforts to gorge on sand food being heavily charged. Mylah filled their unresponsive mouths with her food.

Months into the work, Mylah moved into images of an emergency hospital room. She built an entire environment with nurses and doctors, breathing tubes, and many beds. What brought that necessary intrusion she had experienced into my own body was that Mylah built all this around herself. She herself was inside the ER room she made. She insisted on making this clear to me, in case I would not get it. Did she know how important all this was? Not consciously. But Mylah's self had found a way to communicate what her first months of life had been for her.

Meanwhile, what her parents had requested, that I understand their parenting predicaments, was also happening. This little girl could cuss like a sailor when it was time to go. She took to tossing things at me in her rage. I caught these articles of misgivings, telling her they would stay safe with me. At the same time, she was slowly building a sense of *wanting* to be safe, and to do so might mean that she needed to work with her neurological impulses. As she turned 5, and then 6, Mylah took on board more effort to remain present sooner after an outbreak of aggression. The parents and I worked away at this bruised-up brain, following in the footsteps of Mylah's own signals. Attachment to her parents gradually became more available. Her parents would need to move forward with psychiatric care and whether or not medications were needed in order for Mylah to grasp the complex and overstimulating realities of schooling.

Mylah's use of the toys was crucial, but I needed to remain very alert to her own communications. At that point, my experiences had not pushed me this far into a child's profoundly compromised beginnings. What made me make the commitment to work more deeply with children who had been born addicted? First, again, the parents knew there would be adaptations involved. Our expectations for Mylah were really quite basic. Second, Mylah herself had a brilliant kind of spunk that connected with others, if you could see her behaviors as spunk and not as terrible and in need of fixing. She moved through many shifts in her efforts to include others and to bring them on board as to her needs. At one point, she soundly told me that her daddy was coming and that she could hear his truck pulling up. I knew better than to check at the window. I commented that she wished Daddy would come. She angrily told me no; he *was* coming. Just look! Again I made my comment, broadening it a bit to say that I wished sometimes that he would come, too. She looked as if she was considering throwing a plate of sand at me. I moved closer to provide any amount of regulation to her efforts to reveal her longing. She yelled at me to "shut UP!" I said this must be so tough to feel. Again: "I said BE QUIET!" I agreed that I would be quiet. We settled back down slowly together. Mylah had made a breakthrough in her attachment hunger, finding a way to show me that no amount of fantasy was bringing birth parents back. She was able to make another step toward her adopting mother, finding that her effort had made some sense outside of herself.

Who are we in this probable, or at least, anticipated, mutual state? If I had made a rule that our clinic did not see these highly dysregulated children, Mylah may not have found the way from inside herself to make these precious steps. With some children, we are a vital and small step in a very long trek. We therapists are willing to be dragged into spaces that we would not think about, as if that morning we can say to ourselves, "Today is a good day to become lost together in Annie's abandonment." There have been some days where I am sorting out what is ahead, and I feel myself shrinking as if not to be found as I see the children's needs and volumes of being that I need to be up for this day. We need to know who we are, that we should take these risks. It is as if we may be accused of having gone too far, or of having too many steps missing, when a parent or attorney accuses us of something that, in the relationship with their child, brought up their own triggers. There are dangers. And the healing in this space far outweighs the anxieties we face when we know we are in the place where the child's own fight is to be seen and understood. Surely, some days can bring the unknown closer, and when we are able to make use of that nearness, the heart inhales some recognition.

Working with Parent-Child Fused States

One little boy I worked with, Seth, engaged my heart ahead of my skills, before I ever met him. He had suffered near loss of life within hours after his birth. When I began seeing him, this 6-year-old had all the symptoms of being on the autistic spectrum. He also appeared to be unusually intelligent. But spending time with me seemed almost to create feelings of brutality in him. He threw himself in a corner and wailed, a high keening sound that set my own nerves on edge. I was able to imagine placing myself in a sort of bubble, hearing and sensing him but also able to think. We were simply too close, too skin-to-skin or even muscle-to-muscle, although physically I was perhaps 5 or 6 feet from him. There was a possibility that I was also too far away, since he and his mother still seemed absolutely fused. She was able to read his signs of neediness as a mother reads the signs of a newborn. And why would she have given up that need to do so in herself? She had nearly lost her son even as they had separated. They had hardly become two separate bodies. This, I came to understand, was the sensation of being skin-to-skin. Separation was extremely painful to this child. Both mother and child were terrified that someone would die if separation occurred.

About three sessions into the work, Tuesday afternoons became a unique experience in me. It was as if Tuesdays had their own planet of understanding. I entered a kind of density, like a dark forest. On Tuesdays around lunchtime, I looked around me and here it was again, that deep overgrowth. I felt nervous, questioning my own thoughts. I called myself names, primarily those around being too dramatic. I wanted to get control over this, refuse to admit this as *my* kind of day. But it did not want to leave me. So I began a weekly awareness of feeling into, rather than out of, this density. It seemed to have information for me. As I tracked it, I understood that this forested feeling left me immediately after seeing this one child. I also narrated my experience in consultation. I grew to understand that the pull in him to remain in this forested world was that powerful. I say that it felt "forested." Really, I do not have words for this space that pulled me into this orbit on Tuesday afternoons. I can say that the sensation was real: a blurry, shadowy environment with no other human beings available. And this space carried a dull physical sensation of pain for me, all over my body. Much later I could credit my bodily pain to the physical intrusions that had occurred to keep him alive and which mirrored my own pain at my delivery into this world.

This understanding, such as it was, helped me to construct a rather unique "treatment plan" regarding this child. I obeyed this quixotic polarity of being far apart and close all at the same time. Truthfully, I am not sure I had much choice. But in this way, I managed to stay near Seth and speak with him, while he courageously attempted to realize my presence as separate and simultaneously safe enough. I had him bring some of the things he used as repetitive soothers in his home life into the playroom. We would concentrate on these things, these items that brought Seth into his realities in his home. We sat together closely, which made Seth's body jumpy. During these times, my body felt as though it had been plugged into a wall socket. I sat there nonetheless, accepting his (and my) acute anxiety at my proximity while I focused on a mutual space that I believed we would discover together. It was the mutuality that needed to be built, a filter that he might be willing to make use of. With this as our common language, Seth began to tolerate being separate and not dying.

Alongside Seth's work, his mother and I worked at separation within her. She so needed Seth to be able to go to school, to carry on without her constant presence. At the same time, she was sure that Seth would not tolerate having any distance between them. Her certainty enforced his own certainty, and any separation caused him to collapse. Both mother and son became hyper-aroused when separation threatened, and neither could direct their relationship's way through this. I addressed this with them in the playroom together. Seth agreed that he would allow his mom to sit outside the room, with a heavy piece of string attached between her wrist and his. They agreed that he could test it whenever he needed to, tugging at it to see if Mom responded. Seth also agreed that he would be kind to his mom's wrist. For this session, that is about all Seth did. Test test test. Pull pull pull. During the next session, he actually forgot this thin connection for short periods of time. I ramped up the test: Mom would sit in her car and Seth would see if the string held. With a good deal of relief in me, it did hold. Seth had a rough time during this weaning, because the control of their shared anxiety was shifting, and he felt his mom's lessening presence. We were cautiously creating a new spatial boundary between Seth's body and that of his mother. Seth, I had to hope, would come to rely on the boundary of skin that housed himself.

I met with Mom and coached her on statements she would make; no questions were allowed. Again, Seth's anxiety spiked, and Mom wanted to stop. I seemed to be the breathing of some air between them. I knew Mom needed to believe in Seth's ability to stay alive so that he in turn could go forward toward some distinction of self.

This was a child that demanded, as a part of his survival, that I enter a mutual field with him. Simultaneously, his spikes in anxiety helped me understand how much we were both asking of him. He required me to suffer the painfulness of a newborn who had no capacity to stay alive but to be stock still: no relationship, no otherness. My most effective brace of tolerating this was the gifted consultant person I mentioned earlier and a constant mindfulness to breathe, myself.

Seth became trusting enough to periodically create images in the tray. This trust was a challenge because each effort exposed him. His images were like windows into his fears and body betrayals. Windows separated Seth from his mother's enfolding comfort during the time when a structure all of his own was being assembled. The sand was often too embodying and too provocative for this child's near-death experience. One image that spoke to both of us was of a little toddler in the center of the tray. Around this, in square after square after square, he put up fencing. Later, he removed the child and left all the squares of fencing in place. This image evoked the paradox of life and rigidity. Soon after this, we were talking about his spaces in his home. "I wish I could live inside a house with no windows and doors," he stated. "Then you couldn't get out," was my practical response. "No. Then no one could get *in*." Seth's newborn, critical life trauma would be there in him, to be addressed in many ways as he grew.

Seth had shared a dark shadowy forest time with no dangerous result. From this mutual frightening infant space, he began to tolerate a nearly foreign other: me. He took on some trust in himself as separate, long after this developmental process had passed. As he took my presence in, without the constant repetition of great danger, he began trusting the environment a bit more, and himself in it. Seth grew more able to create images that could be present in a liminal space. His imagination began to access breathing room between himself and his newborn's knowledge. Now an adult, Seth's intelligence works on his behalf. He is very sensitive to others' inner realities. He has challenged himself to go to college and to reveal the style of his thoughts to others. Sharing his thoughts out loud are the very windows that once frightened him. It is likely that Seth will need to revisit and update that life-threatening injury as he continues onward in adult development.

The Therapist's Wounds That Engage

The work with Seth insisted that I readdress my own wounds. I felt pulled too fast and too thoroughly into his work. Such speed of engagement often directs us to look into our own work. I myself had suffered a near-death birth trauma that had physically left its mark in my body. It held residual body pain that demanded that I stay in relationship with its presence, becoming a double-edged voice of both trauma and insight. This injury aligned with Seth's own sensitivities, and we joined up in a shadowy world of newborns and of profound fear. It was difficult for me to swim about in that sensate and nonverbal awareness, tracking regulation on behalf of Seth's arousals. Although I was no longer afraid, Seth's fears felt so familiar to me. My own transference meant becoming more visible with my consult group over what had happened that had been described to me and now what it took to tend to this injury of mine, yet again. I did not particularly want to step into this injury another time. And yet, Seth's thrust into our common experience insisted that I go here, again. And I think this is what transference demands: that we traipse about in our own wounds and injuries more than once and that we credit these wounds with their truths. They are available when we allow this. We consider our task to assist in helping the past to become truly in the past with our clients. In co-transference, we face the opposite: how to make use of our past becoming a presence that offers assistance in healing. And if we can go humbly to those pockets within us, we might access empathy that is not merely using language. Indeed, we embrace a knowledge within us that can and will respond to the child's need to be known and her need to be remembered. We are able to remember because we dare to mind our own experiences in an honest manner, which allows us to accept the child's injuries. And we ourselves are kept safe by another, a supervisor or mentor, minding us.

As children enter their deeper needs, and depend on our presence as other mother-like mentors in their lives to stay so deeply present, we ourselves become exposed. Knowing about this helps us to choose what resources we ourselves need in order to go deeply with the child's own demands. We hear with the sensitivities of a child's own embodied realities. As we carry a child over the terrain that hurt their past, our environments, for a small period of time, seem more doubtful. This is when the two-mindedness is needed, along with the outside other who understands where it is we are in the terrain and in the work.

Ruthie, the child who addressed her invasive brain tumor, creates a ceremony, as she calls it, with native American figures dancing. "They're dancing to the great goddess or something like that." Ruthie's depression has been lifting, and she talks with her parents more about what she can do, given ongoing limitations to her body's energy.

In another four sessions, Ruthie picks up a tennis player. "I was getting really good at this. But right now I can't play like that." She puts the skeleton in the casket and lays two tombstones on it. She seems able to release her sadness and allow the image to hold it now. Then she places a broom upside down, to represent a lit torch, in the center of the death imagery, "So it's shedding light on <u>every</u>thing. Look at all the blood, in imagination; because you can do anything in imagination." It seems as though Ruthie's imagination had greatly frightened her as she absorbed the conversations and the environments of hospital stays. Now her imagination could work to support her, taking the messiness—and the life—of her experiences and laying them into the work of her play.

We spend a few sessions talking about her experiences, about fear, about the future. In Ruthie's final tray, she builds a community. She must place certain known markers in: the grocer's, the church, a school, a lighthouse, a runway. There is an airplane sitting on the runway.

CHAPTER 13

Clare: Transference and Imagination

A long time ago I worked with a small child, 4 years old, whose relatives had accepted care for her. Her parents were very handicapped by their addictions, and the two children had been severely neglected. The degree of chaos that Clare had experienced was shocking. Clare comes into the playroom silently. Her grandmother says she has not ever said much and not to expect much. The world around Clare believes she herself is handicapped.

Her history revealed that Clare had not yet accomplished developmental steps of building trustworthy attachments or representations. To me, this developmental process is almost entirely relationship-ridden. Representations are the feelings that the mother-child dyad create, lose, refresh, ignite, and rest from. These representations move into things: the blanket, a strand of mother's hair, the stuffed rabbit, and things that are stabilizing by their presence, soft and understood by the embodying self of the child. Psychology names these things transitional objects. I think of them as transitional subjects who have been assigned the imaginal life they carry. Lacking the development of this attuned resonance, Clare did not know how to play.

Not Knowing How to Play

When Clare finds the sand, she quietly picks up perhaps a dozen small toothpicks, and one by one, pushes them through the sand. Clare looks somewhat blankly in my direction. I know she needs me to do a certain thing, but it is very difficult to know what she needs. She seems to want me to do something particular that would not threaten her hyperfocus on the sticks. I quietly lift up a small towel in the room and reach out to take her stick offering. "I'll dry them," I say. Clare's shoulders soften just a hair. My choice is coincidently correct. What transpires between us at that moment in time is that Clare could not move toward me at all. She had been dropped off with any number of people, and I am included in the dropping. I join her in her inability to play with my own intention to play someday.

Following this, we wash and dry sticks for about four sessions. For short periods of time Clare might silently walk about the room, looking at the toys, reaching out but not touching. I wonder if the entire arrangement here in this playroom is too "hot." I offer Clare some food, and it seems to frighten her. I narrate that this food could be hers, but it did not need to be hers. In another two sessions, she allows her hunger to risk taking the cereal bar. During this time, I suffer many feelings of needing to speed up, to pull Clare out of this memory that had hold of all of her, to help Clare to find me. I feel inadequate on all counts and don't know what to do. I also feel rage toward the people who had taken away Clare's right to be real to herself. I need support during this time, certainly, and make sure my consultation time is predictable.

Looking back, I believe some of my feelings of anger were protectors so that I might share in Clare's experiences without being overwhelmed by them myself. My transference, my empathy toward Clare's history, pushed me emotionally and somatically. Oftentimes, I felt as though I was caring for a baby in the room. My mothering instincts wanted to make faces and win Clare over to my need to attach with her. This baby-like Clare seemed to have accepted the still face of the parent for an indefinite length of time, and I wanted to push into her space with my intense longing to help. I wanted us both to be alive.

But then Clare starts making her own choices: a bunch of babies in a heap, scary animals who enter but do nothing. We nearly always touch base with some of the washing and drying ritual, more likely near the end of our time together. She adds more communicators to her efforts: holding out the towel for my use, silently putting my hands in the sand and covering them and then washing them. My hands in the sand invoke a terrible sadness in me. Later on, I would understand that feelings like this were from making contact with Clare's own feelings through the sand itself. Clare starts looking at me more, and then she figures out how to smile.

Being Found: The Work of Imagination

The teaching Clare gives to this day is how imagination reopened her capacity to speak from a place of trust. At some point she knew that I had found her and that being seen felt right. Clare was more able to relate with me outside in the open air. I pulled painting supplies and dolls out onto the porch, and we worked together in this airy space. Then she began a game. She would run across a field, maybe 30 feet away from me. Then she would turn and wait for me to crouch low. As she approached me, I would catch her and swing her up and onto her feet, while she laughed. I could sense Clare's captivating focus on just when I was ready to "capture" her. The cues between us flickered like fireflies in the dusk. I myself was remembering the hints and cues of when my own children had been newborns. We did this for maybe 15 minutes every session. We both found it exhilarating. Clare was gaining in her relationship with me. This relationship could easily become nearly giddy, and it was my responsibility to moderate this. Looking back, it may be compared to playing with an infant who does not look away from a cooing adult. The infant continues to get more agitated, smiling and laughing until he begins to cry. We were fitting ourselves together, attuning our knowingness as a duet. The somatic rhythm that this play offered was also important. Clare was learning to trust her own body, and giving in to this embodied self helped her to approach language.

One day she did not run back toward me.

Clare walks back toward me while I watch her for our new signs of connection. Her hands are cupped closed. She comes up to where I am down on my knee and slowly begins to open her hands. "See the bird," she says.

"Ahhh, there is a bird, a beautiful small bird, that's landed in your hand," I respond.

"It's a little baby bird, and it's my friend." This small absolute imaginal presence between us holds feelings in me to this day.

Clare took all of her safety and placed it in her cupped hands that day. And her representation was kept safe, since there were no words that intruded, no efforts to add or subtract the meaning of this for her. Its meaning was the bird itself: There was no room for anything else in that moment. Through the bird, Clare quietly moved from running toward me to an image of a bird flying toward her, to a meaning rich with the containment of what her hands held. This bird, in the emptiness of her hands was *us* too, that co-transference that brought meaning into Clare's self. Her previous meanings of relationship were concretely empty. Her hands on this day were very full.

After this imagination had been caught, Clare went back into the playroom. She cautiously began, very simply at first, to choose miniatures and to put them in the tray. She also brought words into the room with herself. She had somehow, from washing sticks, to running, to a bird, captured her imagination and landed

Clare: Transference and Imagination

a place for her meanings to grow. Together we had moved through immobilizing experiences, to body movement that had its own language for her, to the language of the bird. When she caught this small bird, Clare caught sight of her own meaning, and she got to choose to bring it to me to witness but not to tamper with. It was hers, as any whole symbol is. The image belongs utterly to its creator.

Transference is about relationship at a very deep level. Because children are so porous in their relationship with important others, they bring unedited selves in their approach and in their connectedness. In healthy emotional environments, children make use of their porous realities to "make sense" of what lives between themselves and others. What they pick up on they then make meaning from, and this meaning is stored within memory. Transference will troll these unconscious meanings to find what has been stored and still wants understanding.

Somewhere between transference and the child's observable activities, imagination plays its essential part. Imagination is akin to a moderator, one who sits in the liminal spaces between a this and a that, and weaves meaning that is from the self of the child. An image can be another verb if we let it remain in motion. An image and imagination capture a representation that means something to the child. She feels around, hunting for material like a bird hunts for the twigs to build a nest. Her nest-building will house something she nurses from her own felt interior world. When that is strong enough, she evokes the image to carry what she has found and built, out into an expression. Hopefully, her evocation, her image-making, will speak on her behalf, telling someone outside of her what is so important, what words themselves cannot carry to us, the therapist or parent or teacher. From this creative need inside, images come toward us, with color and juice and the hope that we might better understand the child for her effort. She has invoked a nonverbal language that wants to draw us in with its aliveness. In this effort, words can be flat and not full of enough life. She must let us see this, for we cannot see with flat words. We might just think, and thinking here is not seeing.

At times we are tempted to chuckle at what a child invents in the way of putting words to an experience. I think of this effort as creative work that comes straight out of the child's interior. The child understands that in her world, there is a vulnerability to being so open. There is no logic to this knowing, just a simple recognition that she may not be understood. This comes from experience itself, from the misses and errors of reason that cast shadows over the child's creative meanings.

When a child enters the playroom, he is familiar with toys and with the expectation that these toys will be useful. How useful is somewhat dependent on the therapist's ability to enter imaginatively into the child's own world with that child. And the utility of toys also depends on the depth of the therapist's own capacity to play in the realms of metaphor and image. Here is where imagination lives. It is accurate to say, with Ruth Ammann, that "images are formed, and they become experience, *images* of experience" (R. Ammann, 1991). Images, imagination, dreaming are all from the same creative space within the self.

Access to the Unconscious Through Imagination

Imagination plays a crucial role in its access to the unconscious and in its efforts to communicate what has been hidden. It is the joint between our own inner world and the outer world we inhabit. As such, this unique force provides insights through its use of creative images. Following these images puts us in a more dreamlike state. As in dreams, images are brought to us rather than the ego being in charge. It is this creativity that the child continues to access through play. Reverie lives in this kind of play. And when the child is playing within the awareness of another who regards her play as meaningful, she has the capacity to express truths that may have remained unspoken and unconscious. The other, the witness, enters that reverie with the child. In this style of dreaming together, the relationship serves as a container that might secure something new in its net. The realness of the child, her feelings and perceptions, and her own meanings that she has made are the truths we are waiting to hear from the play. Even though they may remain unspoken in the sense of oral language, these truths might speak clearly and to the point within the play and the relationship itself.

If adults have discounted or overridden the child's truths, these feelings are stored away. Having felt that hurt, the child's truths may continue to stay unconscious in the child's implicit meaning-maker. However, a therapist trained in mending through play tracks the images and comprehends the story that the child conveys. The therapist is charged with some amount of consciousness while the child is charged with trusting the relationship in order to create out of his own truths.

Imagination and Maria

Another child, Maria, was stern in her exposure of her images. What was it she meant when she told me she had been watching a small dragon in her trees at home? And when I asked Maria if her mom knew of this dragon, her huffy response was "Are you kidding me?! Of course not! I've only told you!" I knew I had injured Maria's relationship with me by becoming suddenly concrete. And we set about repairing that. What had she meant for me to understand? It was not merely about dragons at all. It was more deeply about trust, that the reality which the two of us shared came from the reality of imagination, and that in this environment, Maria needed me to walk beside what kept her connected to herself: some creative hot-tempered force. And she insisted that I be trustworthy in carrying her images, even when I stumbled a bit.

Maria was intelligent to the point of exhausting those around her, and her own intensity gauge utilized much imagination and story to maintain any pacing for herself. At age 6, she had already taken to "running away" as her parents called it, and "disappearing" as she referred to it. This disappearing act entailed many parts, like chapters to a book, into which Maria could climb and let go of a bit of the pressures of being her own self. She could not construct how impossible it was for her to have so many ports of information coming into her brain and into her psyche. She had to make use of her body and her ability to imagine her own reality. In this sense, Maria's intelligence was not helpful to her in her younger years. It pushed at her so hard when her brain was not strong enough to balance itself, to take pauses, and to think thoughts that might calm her. She could not keep up with how many feelings ran within her all the time. Running an imaginary life gave Maria internal rooms to withdraw into. When that was not enough, she separated from too much parent engagement by disappearing, "running away" long enough to reconnect internally.

Intelligence will attempt to make order of all this input, but in a young child's brain, it is not successful for any long period of time. Maria turned me toward her need to disappear and away from running away. My learning curve was obvious to both her and me since I became anxious about her parents' reactions to their definitions of her behaviors. And, truthfully, are we not the midwives to this difference in definition? It was not yet safe for Maria to be gone alone and without parent awareness, no matter what you want to call this. But, neither was it safe for Maria to feel unknown in her profound efforts to balance intelligence and empathic feelings with the difficulty in understanding her needs. Simply put, she did not feel safe internally and she had no idea how to let that be known.

Clare: Transference and Imagination

Maria managed to demand that her parents, who were divorced, both come in to see me, with she herself being the moderator. I was concerned about how this might go, but agreed to it. We prepared for this time with our heads together. She drew scenes on a paper that might give them a view of her own interior map. Some of what she put on the map was confrontational, and I let it be, knowing that I would also be in the room. Maria began this session letting her parents in on some of the pressures she carried. I remember well the respect that carried me through this odd parent consultation.

Today Maria is a play therapist. Who she is, and who she was as a child, continue to inform her. Her personal experiences are a pulse, a baseline for her professional information gathering. She sees hyperactively intelligent children who are difficult to find.

We talked earlier about the hunger in the child to be seen and to be known. The interspace between two people is where the child is continually heading out from, building a personal self with a personal ego that will hold steady as the human being develops. We might say that the ego is that aspect that continues to develop an individual, that restores and refreshes the meanings that make "me" the "me" that I am. The toys that are chosen in the effort to express "me" participate as images in the field of experiences. In this way, I am still safe. I am still the child that is learning to separate from who you think I am. My creative play instills the toys into my experience, laying it out like a dream or series of dreams. They are of me, but keep me a little hidden. Remember the little girl in chapter 10, Mona, who made jagged teeth with her name on them. When her mom came to pick her up, she saw the drawing on the floor and asked Mona about it. "Oh," said Mona, "those are big hills." Nothing dangerous at all. She simply was not ready to expose her adoptive mom to her own hidden terrors and her intense feelings.

Imagination in play is powerful. Through it the child collects trust. When the therapist continues to enter into the creative efforts of the child's play, without use of logic, remedy, or solution, the child continues to push on, toward that shared space, and toward where injuries occurred. The imagination is the heft within the play, that inspiration which reveals the child's own meanings, while being held with grace.

I recall at age 3, an afternoon when a number of farmwomen gathered out in the sun with their iced tea to share some stories. They were each sitting properly but relaxed. I recall noting their postures and feeling a desire to be like them, to join with them. I remember the feeling of comfort that they shared. The tones of their laughter and their storytelling pulled me toward becoming one of them. Wrapped in my sensation of well-being, I pulled up a milk bucket and sat down. The trouble was, my 3-year-old brain did not register which side of this pail would be a chair, and I fell in, bottom first. I was devastated and enraged as every one of them laughed heartily at me. My anger seemed to only engage their laughter further. My own goal, of joining and being like them, completely disappeared. What makes this memory significant here is that I had been utterly engaged in an imaginal space, like a tea party, in which I would suddenly *be* one of the adults that I admired. That imagination was flowing from within me, wanting an image to become an experience. Inside me, it was a possibility. Instead, I would hold onto it along with a myriad of other internally snapped images that would need sorting at an older age. I would wonder if these image-making events were collisions between the creative images of a child and their surprisingly concrete events.

My own experiences help me to better understand the workings of the imagination as a liveliness that yearns to ease the gaps between the child's knowing and the adult wanting to know. Between a "you" and a "me" is an intermediate realm, and imagination is the entity that serves both of us and moves us to a shared knowing. In these states of reverie, we are "us." The play is the child's, and the attuned other that allows the play's realness is the therapist. Who would want to enter this field and kick the bucket into concrete reality? Let's not.

Relational Space as Imaginal Space

Let's draw the map of where we have traveled. The relationship of attunement and mirroring pulls the child and the therapist toward right-brain-to-right-brain wiring, toward the trust that is primal in its integrity and not conscious in its language. As these two people move closer to one another and into the implicit world of meaning rather than rational thought, they approach co-transference. The two move toward both mutual recognition and toward resistances that may exist as protectors from old hurts. Both of these, the toward and the away from, are surfacing in right-brain-to-right-brain connection. The therapist has agreed to risk his well-informed hold on his reality (not their shared reality) in order to connect with this child.

The child, as she feels the approach of care, emotional availability, and trust, approaches meanings that have been arrested. As the child feels this growing resonance, she moves inward toward her truths. Again, we call this dependency. From this interior space, the child chooses her own best language: Poetry? Singing? Sand images? Excitement that knows no bounds? How will she speak as she adjusts to the resonance of another? Transference creates an opportunity now, a space from which the child speaks in her authentic voice. "Speaking" is the imagination. The toys are the words and paragraphs, while the relationship is the carrier that enlivens things and turns them into subjects. These words are selected by the child's imagination. They are not driven by a need to communicate thoughtful descriptions that help one person to build a shared image: The shared image is what comes into the tray and is held by the therapist. Transference is the shared space; imagination carries the conversation.

I say that one person is playing. That is not quite accurate. One person is guiding the play with her imagination hard at work. The other is playing in the field of the child's perceptions, holding steady with the assignments that are given to him, even assignments that he cannot bear, that reveal themselves in embodied states. Imagination is the bridge, the feeling and the dreamed embodiment that becomes an image and holds still with the meaning it presents. It remains full of life as long as it is needed. Imagination makes the choices of miniatures that must enter the tray, and with each entry, the child ponders, wonders why that one showed up, and then tells the story that is found there. Imagining brings about meaning from within the child.

In working with young children, this imagination world and co-transference fully interact. The child might move toward these rich images, but she counts on the therapist moving with her as the indicator of inter-trust, interdependency. In the arena of transference, we are being called to create bridges where pieces of being human were not built strongly enough. As we stay at attention in these interspaces, the child sees into our presence. This seeing into is that primitive knowing that runs through the mutual fields of infant/parent, child/therapist.

Children still have access to unconscious forces through their porous filters. By the time we are adults, we have clipped and sewn many more rigid filters over this arena we call the unconscious. It can become a transgression to pull material out of this space, as if we are thieving from ourselves. For children, however, this space still reigns with power. Its messages reveal themselves in metaphor, play, "out of the blue" narrations, and dreams. Sandplay welcomes these energies and makes use of their features in story-building. The unconscious carries our own experiences mixed up with the charged feeling tones and throbs of others. There has been very little ownership of what got thrown into the overall design. If some of the fragments are painful, the child does not necessarily question why they hurt. When pain becomes overwhelming, the child will dissociate from that area, causing an overburden that is not quickly named or sorted as to whom it belongs.

The Therapist's Assignments

In playing within the child's implicit meanings, we add to the meaning the child has been creating. We are not to change or interpret the meaning; our own regard for the child's images enhances the child's efforts so that she might own something new. Something energetic has been sent out, received, and returned, and in this return the child is able to know. Recall Andy's finger-drawn map in the tray. Andy tells me the child "will go home." In that play, Andy could begin to imagine a map that sent him back home. But he did not yet have the stamina to carry out the feeling of what he imagined. It is the attuned engagement of mothering: The infant gives out from within what cannot be digested. The mother absorbs this, and her digestion of its meanings are now palatable. She returns it to the infant in digestible form.

Imagine for yourself the degrees of trust, and indeed, of faith, that the child obeys in order to bring us into their inner world of the implicit. Over and over, our work demands that we honor the unconditionally hard work that is relationship. The toys are simply a medium through which faith is built, and through which experience achieves a face. When the child experiences the adult's presence in a shared feeling state, the toys have done their work. It is the journey from the inner implicit world in the child, into an image that imagination has created, that leaps into the arms of the mutual field: the transference. In the transference, the child *knows* he no longer carries his injuries alone. Someone else is present in the implicit reality, and is standing by as implicit memory re-opens, and then refreshes itself. He *knows* some other being has submitted to an inner reality that seemed intolerable in its unknowingness. And now it is doable. This is at the heart of healing: Our being alive is doable.

Imagination, Remembering, and Being Remembered

Remembering and imagination are first cousins, and they live in nearby realities. They help one another in taking care of the child's true sense of reality and of the self, until such time as greater strengths evolve within the child. Even then, however, these relatives hang steady, keeping witness to the interior growth of the child. It is imagination, with remembering at its side, that sustains becoming a creative adult and that holds the two-sided coin of work as play and play as work.

Authenticity, that reality of being genuine to oneself, is the deep result of trust. When I am recognized, I settle into coming into myself. My self-ness is the result of the back-and-forth resonance of the two of us dancing together, fitting ourselves together, and daring to understand one another in this fitting. The child experiences herself as separate because she has been unconditionally regarded within this mutual relationship. Relationship and its trust are created and then refreshed constantly in the mending process. When relationship is strong enough, small mistakes on the part of the play therapist can be forgiven and can work to strengthen the child's confidence, as when Jake called me on my weak response to having real fear of the dragon. Children move toward authenticity as they experience a consistent presence that says, "I see you." Co-transference has enabled both child and therapist to endure temporarily shared wounds. In passing through these old mine fields, the child embodies the belief that "I am still alive, and for that matter, so are you!" Young children in their self-centering often believe that their anger, and even more so,

Clare: Transference and Imagination

their infant rage, will tear apart the person they are leaning on. That lean may have been very threatened, as many times the need to depend on someone went unnoticed.

The rituals the child obeys from internal guidance in her play are the actors in imagination. The creator feels about and comes out with a storyline that communicates to the witness what it is that is wanted, and even where to find it within the child's memories. The request, sometimes the plea, "Will you remember me?" asks the therapist to accompany the child along this internal pathway to a reference point in the child's self. This centering reference point might be covered for protection; it may be nearly missing in action but not quite. To discover and to recover this centering point, an other is required for the child's self. This is not a thinking place at all, and those who want to believe it is may be unwilling to credit the child's own inner resources. Children who still believe in the reliability of adults will reach out to nearly any adult with the felt sense of potential trust.

In working with children who have been hurt, there are layers upon layers of unintegrated needs and meanings the child has assigned to her experiences. In this effort to make meaning, children are quite available to adults who are trying to understand. Meaning-making wraps a skin around one's experiences in order that they not remain fragmented and too frightening to be located. We adults are the witnesses and the mirrors to each child's own meanings, which, coming from the child's own perceptions, take a little time to understand. Many times, however, adults approach understanding through their own pre-established models. Models might be how parents think children are supposed to behave, what the child must learn regardless of their history, or behavioral cognitive techniques that work best with diagnostically identified children. The reality is that the clearer we adults can be in establishing an empty space that greets the child (not merely the challenges on the intake form), the more the child will be able to listen internally for what wants comprehension.

The children whose lives and whose work say far more than I can narrate are heroic. At the same time, they are hunting for the person who will support the deepest aspects of being human, being whole. Many times I have wondered if the work I witnessed would hold in the child. After many years, when some of the children I had seen between the ages of 3 and 7 were now becoming adults, I could see the traces, like dreams dreamed long ago, of where we had traveled together to find them. In this small community, the child and I would both feel uncomfortable when a parent or grandparent would excitedly point me out and insist by their tone that we say something. I could see that the child barely remembered me. Maybe he barely wanted to remember me. I had been absorbed into that right-brain meaning-maker, and it was troublesome to bring me up. Sort of like bringing up one's babyhood to an audience. The child's faith in me had become useful. His history of play with some person who offered a lot of toys was now ordinary. The child's understandings had moved from an interior world, toward trust, into imagination, then into play, and finally into experiences that were the child's own subjective, ordinary world. My faith in the child had taught me about movement on a map, about breathing when one is lost, about consciously loving another person and wanting for them what we all deserve, and about traveling together to find this opus.

Part IV
Supervision

Chapter 14

Supervision: Faith and Doubt

I recall spending time in South Dakota with the Lakota people. An old (not in age so much as in experience with Spirit) medicine man taught me many things simply by watching his interactions and remaining open to his path of depth. At times he made seemingly sudden decisions that outwardly looked random and harsh. Following the implicit meaning of the spirit of relationship that he obeyed always brought sense to the seeming randomness. I understood better the value and the apparently hard line that trusting the truth brought about. This man had been mentored from a very young age, brought up in the traditions of his people's medicine way. And it took faith in this man to really discover the larger context of an event. What we might see was the situation itself. Under and within was a deeper meaning. My gratitude for the trust this elder put in me still grows in me. The medicine man demanded that people's relationships between self and Self, or Spirit, as he referred to this, was clear-sighted, and that intentions were honorable.

Do we approach our child clients with such regard, with clean and honorable intentions? Or do we find ourselves to be instead the braver or the smarter of the two in the healing relationship? If our braver need is reinforced by our own access to diagnoses, and possibly the definition of best practice, we have already deserted some degree of faith in the child's self. In order to find ourselves in the claws of transference, we will have had to submit to a polishing off of ego positions. At the same time, enough ego is required in order that we maintain the small footprint that defines us as individuals, as we may find ourselves in a chaotic mishmash of feelings that were not there before, when all we had to deal with was our own little ego.

These are the undercurrents we bring into supervision. As we therapists track our child clients, we ourselves must be tracked, kept track of. Therapists feel both faith in ourselves, and also authentically bring our doubts to this structured time each week. As we are the pivot points in relational strata with the children we serve, our supervisors are fulcrums with whom we test our professional knowledge, our internal instincts, and our connections between self and other. We come out of hiding to reveal our own relationship with the child through a wider lens that mirrors the faith we have in the work itself. When we approach humbly, and humanly, our mistakes and our appreciations, we breathe in the understandings we have sought.

Most of us do not have the native medicine path or other alternate routes that often mentor in the ways of trust and faith. And yet, to keep tracking through the diagnosis, past the prepared plan, heading on into the heart of the child's need, mentorship is needed. This return to the fullness of relationship enables us to enter into the child's world and be the quiet, unwavering other who remains receptive to the child's "playing alone in the presence of" us (Winnicott, 1971). Tracking the "us" *and* the "me," we bring all of this into supervision. A skilled supervisor will have sensed when a deepening state is coming into the playroom and will be prepared to contain the therapist's own activated and primarily unconscious realities.

At times we wonder if supervision is needed once we are licensed. The initial point of supervision is not to access hours toward a goal. It is about being neophytes in a task that requires oversight. The hours that are required toward licensing demand that we push ourselves in our professional learning. Being initially inexperienced, and being witnessed ourselves, these requirements will find us a little more astute in our awareness regarding children. We are granted 2, maybe 3 years, to build that astuteness. Yet, each child brings us the challenge of making use of what we know while listening for that child's unique internal map, and that child's best capacity to reveal and communicate what is being asked of us. If we are committed to our personal and professional growth and the deepening grasp of relationship, honesty, presence, and healing, we will experience each new child pushing us past the comfort of what we thought we knew. This is as it should be. Standard requirements provide a structure behind which live the context of the relationships we travel within. Enough structure allows deeper surrender to the unconscious needs that each child carries about. While realizing their legal commitments, the interrelationship of supervision, consultation, and play therapy embraces the heart of the work.

Being Found as the Therapist Self

Supervision is a central connecting joint in working with children. When a supervisor has not had experiences of being found in the mutual field with her own mentor, she will not be able to trust the therapist who is struggling with transference. It is crucial to have had those experiences in which a mentor has trusted this current supervisor's own efforts to build a pathway through the hurt and tangle of a child's pain. It is always this trust in another's efforts that apprentices professionals. When one has been treated with kindness and curiosity, the centering awareness makes use of those experiences in becoming a guide with others.

Here is the crucial importance of supervision. The supervisor is charged with a more alert wiring-up to the therapist, a task I refer to as connecting at the hip. Knowing enough of the terrain of the unconscious, the supervisor assures right-brain-to-right-brain attachment, and unconscious to unconscious. In this particular relationship, the supervisor carries a parallel two-mindedness that the therapist sustains in the playroom. Images and sensations express shared meanings while the two venture into the child's expressed work and the therapist's own responses and dreams of that work.

When we therapists are strapped to the hip of a guide, we are able to lower ourselves into the experiences of the child, to offer recognition. The meaning of recognition is "an awareness that something perceived has been perceived before"; "to know or identify from past experience or knowledge"; "an acceptance as true or valid" (American Heritage Dictionary, 1992). Perception lies in the realm of implicit feeling states that haunt the child's experiences and remain invisible and nonverbal. Recognition of the child's past dangers gradually releases the child from the harm done. The vehicle of this work is the transference and our own willingness to arrive here in the hurt spaces of the child, to witness the validity of non-verbalized experiences, and to carry the child toward her own empowerment and validation of her memories. Shut off memories reenter, bringing with them energy that had been closeted. In moments that release energies, the therapist might feel overwhelmed and disorganized. Transference is most likely in these times, as the child reaches out, again and again, to have these frightening experiences seen and transformed.

The Rawness of Hope

Children come into their work with a raw hope and a scarcity of filters. The more vulnerable reality of simply being a child gives some of this rawness its character. We experience their hope in safely leaning into someone else, and it moves us toward a sense of response and responsibility. As we go closer to their gravitational pull of need, we are also moving more closely into strong feelings within ourselves. These might include purposefulness, urgency, hopelessness, doubt, and above all, love. In working with adults, the adult client's own defenses help us to take it a bit more slowly. I have always found myself deeply in the work with a child very early on, while my work with new adult clients has often been paced by the adult's original push/pull. And my own longing for the child's authentic story to be clarified also thrusts me heavily into the work. Supervision and consultation for my work have always remained present, and I have had the blessings of aware and curious people to work with.

Working in co-transference may well be the most demanding space in working with children. Therapists are asked to witness what within a child needs to be understood and where that child wants to be heard from the perceptions and feelings she has brought to bear. When a child has been hurt, or illness is demanding that the child negotiate realities not ideally meant to be in childhood, there comes to be an overload of feelings with little comprehension or organization. These become the moments during which we waver in recognizing the child's experiences. Yet, approaching as closely as possible to understanding their language of need, we are urged to trust the child's process of healing. The truth is that the child is pushing into any of our own unresolved experiences as we fit ourselves to her own need to be understood. We will stop short of understanding if we stop at the crossroads of our own undigested pain–and call that stop by the child's name rather than our own.

Part of the nature of transference, in working with the young, is that children have no strong internal thermometer that knows when to turn down the heat when they are hot. So the therapist suffers the burden of both being in the heat and watching over the child's own temperatures. A full-on unconscious need from the child can feel like a dragon in the room. We often feel unprepared for this volley of intensity. The added requirement in working with children is that we understand the probability of this child's level of trust in us, and therefore the potential presence of the dragon.

Transference with a child may be more available because of the child's less-rigid defenses and her incentive to be seen. The shadowy aspect of working with children is the permeability of their defenses. When a child embarks on her healing journey, we will meet her in this more permeable landscape. We must be ready with some self-awareness. We must have done a hefty degree of our own work so that we are able to discern when our triggers step into the shared space between a child and ourselves.

The child's implied realities are the child's own important communications. It is essential that the therapist use the most genuine gestures that arise from his own faith in the child, himself and the work. The child crosses a threshold to find the therapist present. With that, the child has the option to make an Us. He continues to build his story, his own myth, using this mutuality that lives in the room.

In supervision, the therapist and the supervisor listen to the child's "news," his stories, together. Listening in this context includes both attending to images the child uses and the feelings in the room. When a felt sensation is missing, the supervisee may be a more vulnerable container to the child's work because these feelings are *some*where. Most commonly the therapist is carrying the affect that the child is still not feeling secure enough to reveal. The challenge is in whether or not the therapist is aware of this. Oversight is required here. The supervisor stays in touch with herself while at the same time maintaining enough space from the therapist's own feelings and reactions to listen to the child's realities through the eyes and heart of the therapist. The supervisor also attends to her own interior responses: How is she being affected by the therapist's presence and delivery of story? What is the therapist's body language, tone of voice, facial expressions? Does the supervisor feel the vitality and vividness of the child's own work and how that work enters this container? This is meta-communication: listening both to the material and for the context of all the relationships being brought into this container, including, most crucially, the child. The supervisor comes to know each child that her supervisees carry. She is truly engaged in a field that shares unconsciousness, and her task is to help make use of this mutual field. The supervisor is the mentor who can consistently bring the therapist to center, to listening: listening for the child's path, listening for one's own path that is aroused because of the therapist's care. The same context that we bring to each therapy hour is what the supervisor brings to the supervisory hour.

The Supervisor as Co-regulator

The supervisor co-regulates the work the therapist contains. Another listening ear attends to the work. The child's stories, sensations, and questions are conscientiously available and are held by the supervisor. Enquiries are an active dynamic in supervision and in consultation, urging therapists to retain curiosity for the child's work. The therapist will be called to link up with the child's nonverbal wounds. The wounds were often created when the child's own development was most vulnerable. It is only logical that this therapist will experience a good amount of the child's wounding, and the rawness of its origins. The supervisor must know about this territory and must appreciate the therapist's tolerance for carrying the child's pain all the way through to healing. Here is the pivot of faith, not blind faith, but real faith in the therapist's integrity. The supervisor offers to the therapist what the therapist will safely offer to the child.

What if the therapist is off-center in understanding the child? When we are in the shared empathic state with our child clients, it becomes very difficult to know what belongs to the child and what belongs to the therapist.

As a supervisor for many years, I have witnessed play suffer particularly in beginners less aware of the depth of children's play. I recall entering a playroom shortly after the child had been picked up. Sand was everywhere; the room was shouting its overload. It was all I could do to not act out and shout at the therapist! My own internal confrontation of the spillage, at nearly every level, needed an outlet. I calmed myself, then told the therapist to include photos of the floor and the toy shelves. I made notes and became very clear about what needed addressing before this child came again. The therapist would need to go backward into trust again, before proceeding. This remained a constant focus in the supervisor/supervisee work.

Sand everywhere can at times be the work. The agreement to hold a mess in the container of the therapist and the room can be important. So it is not the concrete appearance of disheveled sand or toys that is the only attention. Rather, of great concern is the new therapist who falls prey to believing the "free and protected space" means freedom to create chaos. Subtleties such as this are what separate the witnessing therapist from the unaware therapist. These disparities in the physical environment point toward the emotional/felt environment. Good supervision entails helping the supervisee to face the boundaries of what she can contain honestly and with clarity, and to explore how she experiences her own parameters. Building this honest and genuine exploration permeates the relationships she develops with her child clients.

There are times a therapist reviews the images from several weeks of a child's work and is in such awe that the truth of the child has become elevated to the divine child archetype. The therapist has transmuted the child's pain into some type of saintly aura. In these times, the human needs of the child have been overstepped. This is a more subtle boundary-breaker. We have a right and a goal to be able to understand the archetypes at play in symbolic work with children. At the same time, we best not travel in this space if we cannot carry the humanness of the child in our own hearts and minds. This is vital. It is one thing to be a mirror in the child's inner world. It is quite another to see one's own inflated needs in that mirror. And the supervisors and consult groups we choose must be a part of going into co-transference spaces. These others in our own lives are the mirrors we trust so that we continually clarify whose labor we are in.

Faith and Doubt

Our own injuries make us vulnerable to the injuries of others. When the play therapist's own triggers are activated, we are in our own right-brain feeling centers. If we had not earlier worked these triggers in our own containers, the raw work with children will likely find them. The result for the therapist is a sense of dislocation or disorganization. Fumbling for meaning, she looks into the space between herself and the child. This is holy ground, and the experienced supervisor will enter this space with authority and compassion. By not denying the child's pain, the therapist is able to bring the nurturance the child is so hungry for. The supervisor who can walk the distance between relationships as a witness, will also see the therapist's own woundedness. With this support, the therapist's own connections with the child remain in their dynamics as she herself ignites some light of change, with understanding and compassion. The names of symptoms that might keep the therapist linked to reason return to their context and where they live: in the story of the child. The supervisor watches over unconscious and potential enactments, ready to be stern and conscientious on behalf of the relationship that is in its molting process: that of the child and the therapist.

The injuries that surface can lead us to enact our anger, our own abandonment, and even our past abuse, with our supervisor. Having supervision that understands this experience when it happens is crucial. We best not believe we can go here alone. Therefore, as a prevention, we must check the containers that keep our work safe to assure that we ourselves are being attended. I will not forget a very intelligent, skilled consultant I had for many years. At one point I knew my care for a child was so great that I was losing my ability to understand the child's own best steps in her immediate future. I took this confusion to my consultant. At first, she seemed to want to use her great intelligence to save *me*. My anxiety increased, as time seemed to shrink. I needed help, and I had no idea how to even point to it. But I was able to say to this person, "You're on the wrong track. This child needs both of our attention, and I am lost. Help me out!" This very gifted person looked a bit shocked, recentered herself, and the two of us recovered my own attachment to my safety net. And she thanked me for my honesty. My trust in this woman as my consultant doubled. I knew that she could hear my confusions and have the faith in me I needed, while at the same time she could align me with her containment of my work as needed. These supervisors and consultants are hard to come by. And they are vital. Transference, in its higher levels of charged mutuality, has the real danger of pulling us into a shared space that truly belongs to the client's own use, even while we share that space for a leg in the journey.

The supervisor is the go-between that helps us understand, through experience, how to bring our own structures back into the human connection–back into the places where injuries reveal themselves and beg for the relationships that will mend them. If we have committed energy to our client, we will inhale sharply, test our supports, and head in. Jung states somewhere (as does the Bible) that we cannot relate to others unless we have that relationship in place ourselves. And so transference is as a welcoming hand in that we ourselves evaluate how far we have come in this interior structure of the self, how much strength we have in our interior, and what are the states of our own injuries.

False Knowing

As a mentor, I have witnessed times when a therapist seems to be rather suddenly full of confidence in his decisions, when 2 weeks ago he had reported anxiety and confusion. The therapist had changed his position and had wanted the child to say in words what the child was experiencing in the session. The new confidence of the therapist, a belief that he knows what the problem is for the child, might now overstep the boundaries of the parent or caregiver by naming his professional thoughts in a manner that uncloaks his own inflated beliefs. He has become the specialist, the one whose education helps him to figure out family systems while the members of the system who have lived the experiences are right there in front of him. What has caused this erratic inflation of his self-assuredness?

When the inflation of assumed wisdom strikes, we are gripped in the claws of very big meanings of our own for which we deny the need for any outside checking. Because the illusion has originated through honest insights, there is little emphasis that we should check out loud on these feeling states. This is open ground in which to make any number of errors. The inflation might easily and unthinkingly put us as the best parent the child has, the best understanding agent. The original need for expression of *our* self, the therapist, steps out beyond the child's imagination. Even though hard to spot, our own egos are driving us. The imaginative field that gave us our understanding is withering. Imagination aspires to express the self. Inflation pulls us into what the ego needs, and in doing so, we are no longer the alchemical assistants to the child's creations. We will have lost the trust and the faith in the child's own healing. We are sure we can do what we really wanted to do all along: Save the child. This will always be an impossibility.

Inflation here is often due to having likewise heard the child's own truths within ourselves. However, our container for these truths which resound so succinctly with our own truths is not strong enough. We have not stopped long enough to name our own feelings and instead rush out with a new thought that has not stabilized. Our own swollen sensations save us from further pain in ourselves that would have been due to the transference within the child's work. Our own voice becomes driven by the ideal half of what has been triggered. The painful half is deserted.

Any number of therapists have allowed the child to take toys physically from the room, particularly miniatures that had been the child's own charged feeling representatives. When this has happened, the work has not been kept in the container that the therapist must hold, and the crack in the containment can easily endanger the child's process. Sometimes I have gone in to observe, in order to check in on the therapeutic relationship. I have seen a kind of giddiness that lets me know the therapist is approaching his own limits. Here the danger of enactment increases. One such experience was the therapist telling the 7-year-old about her own childhood as it related to the child's hungry needs. Another was the excitement in the therapist that the child finally killed the evil sorcerer, when, in fact, the therapist's definition of what that toy represented had become too diagnostic. In supervision, the therapist remembered that in times past, the evil sorcerer had also represented protection.

The supervisor requires a verbal commitment between herself and the therapist when the therapist is vulnerable to enactment. One example when the therapist has become involved in a disorganized family system is to tell the therapist that no emails or communications may leave the clinic until the supervisor's eyes have been on them. When the relational world seems to be heating up with its demands, the supervisor is charged with helping to pace the heat, keeping enough warmth while at the same time burning no one. The therapist experiences the relief that something very central is happening. Often, there is also increased stamina in the containment of the therapist because he recognizes that someone is caring for him in this crossing. And with this relational link in place, the therapist can safely go a bit further than he may have, continuing to find the child in the child's own experiences, finding the child within a system that may not be able to find the child.

Many of us have been told to separate our work from the client's. And this is solid education and advice. But being told something does not stop our own triggers from firing off and our own pockets of hurt seeing a chance to be noticed. Working in co-transference is nearly inevitable when working with children. We are easily pulled toward the child's painful story and then find ourselves urgently wanting to provide some safety. When we see a child who is hurting so deeply, it is truly human to hear the inner voices that demand that we offer something more, more than the anticipated therapeutic relationship, to bring about the care we understand they need. Being told to not go to sacred ground may work for a while. At some point, however, the sheer care of another puts us in the place where our own shadows show up. Our choice and our commitment becomes about *us,* ultimately: How do we ourselves constantly approach awareness and compassion toward that which dances us? In this conundrum, the supervisor holds the key to keeping the therapist in resonance with the child's own pace, while both therapist and mentor carry the child's work toward a conclusion that includes safety.

The Strength of the Unconscious

I worked with an intern who was herself in therapy. At one point, the child's session had been interrupted by an abusive parent. Although she acted appropriately, the intern accused me of being unavailable, which had put the child and herself in danger. Her accusations were sharp and aggressive. For months we remained aware and active about her hostility toward me and her belief that I had been at fault. She did not trust me. My efforts at being her supervisor were fraying. Near the end of her internship, she began having some very violent dreams. She worked on those in her private therapy. Her own childhood abuse broke into her consciousness and into our work. In this, she realized her accusations of my ineptness were the result of her own very young terrors vis-a-vis a long-ago parent. There was enough safety in our relationship that an implicit memory entered and demanded full-on to become known. She had absorbed the child's molestation and felt its approach within her own awareness. The invasion of privacy and safety had been identical in its implicit memory. The intern's past had become present.

When we have not owned our work through personal therapy and good consultation/supervision, we are at risk of doing harm to the child's trust. Transference can appear through having felt uncomfortable, sleepy, or bored. We might dissociate and leave the relationship to its own dance, with little awareness available. When we allow the child to break toys or make messes that are not contained, we have stepped away from our own awareness. These are the interactions that an experienced and alert supervisor notices. The discussion with the therapist will include these observations and the means that will refocus the therapeutic relationship on the child's needs. Ungoverned transference lets the child feel our own unconscious messiness, our implicit memories which are surfacing as they match the child's pain that is in the room. The

Supervision: Faith and Doubt

end result of remaining unconsciously engaged and unavailable in the child's process is that we break boundaries.

Even with training and structures in place, gray areas exist between the supervisor's tasks and the therapist's private therapy work. When transference ignites, this area becomes murky with questions about whose tasks are whose. One filter to use is that the focus in supervision remains intent on the child's work and the relationship between therapist and child. When the therapist comes to supervision with material that has triggered the therapist's transference, the supervisor facilitates sorting out the messiness that transference has unleashed. A greater challenge, however, is when the therapist's own transference includes the supervisor in its grip. She may be playing out a good or a not-good parent, or a competitive aspect of the therapist that needs to prove himself right. The supervisor directs the discussion toward the child's work and into where experiences in the playroom roused the therapist's triggers. Dynamic materials between therapist and supervisor are in service to the work the therapist carries. The supervisor is charged with monitoring the work in the playroom. The therapist's private therapy plays an important, less visible, role in the therapist's own ignited dynamics.

Being in therapy ourselves is a prophylactic that captures some of our own unconscious blips and break-ins, and provides insight and charting of our material. This material is where we can become lost when the child chooses to trust our efforts. Our failures in relationship may be shared with the failures the child is carrying. A good consultation group, which houses other therapists who are working in a similar depth approach with symbols and metaphors, is also worth a great deal.

The unconscious has its own strength and energy. It demands that we therapists continually address our own ego stamina to help withstand the forces of an unknown environment. We are not pushing out or overcoming the great importance of ego presence.

Instead, we form a different relationship that tolerates discovery and patience while we sit in the presence of a child's hurt and need. We are taught a sufficient outline that enables each of us to continue on into energies that let us know, while we ourselves learn to track, there is something tracking us, letting us know from a place of unknown. The child lives so close to this realm that the use of sand, art, and metaphor pull from this field and as the child emerges, he moves toward us in dreamlike images. When we are on a firm interior ground, we accept the donations of the bent twig, the hoof mark in the mud, or the sound in the dark that the child's unconscious throws our way. We have a choice: Are we willing to submit to experiences that our Western culture often finds impractical, in order to learn about a reality that is always available? In this space, we move from implicit memory toward building a sacred space of safety so that linkages between two people will occur. Receptivity in the therapeutic relationship, which has few words, holds what was unbearable while it becomes nameable. As the child can feel and think about what has been unconscious, they become *my* experience, and they are *me*. The child's experiences are capable of ownership because someone stepped into this child's perceptions and saw the child with these feelings, and no harm came to the child while having them. This is at the foundation of being *found*.

When we can truly sense the inner life of another, we link together. "Two separate entities, two individuals, become linked as one connected system when subjective experience is attended to, respected, and shared" (Siegel, 2017). These connections, by way of attunement, integrate what could not enter and now does. Siegel goes on to articulate that it is this integration that ultimately creates self-organization, from the inside out and from the bottom up. This is also the notion of the whole being more than the sum of its parts.

The myths and metaphors of the spirit are the stories of the heart. We cannot make the experience happen. It cannot be run at, forced, or induced. "It is a form of grace—through the desire for wholeness" (Churchill, 2021). Ultimately, the healing we hunt for is inside ourselves. I recall a child of 4 years, who made use of the old myth of Pegasus. When she allowed me to look upon her work during its most dangerous passage, I was commanded to only look through a mirror, and the great danger was a very large snake. One could argue that she knew the myth of Medusa and Pegasus. She did not, at least not in her consciousness. Yet, in her need for healing, she had descended into a universal myth. She followed its course as she brought to me the decisive manners through which to face the dread of her experiences. To look upon them directly, and upon her, was in itself a repetition of her abuse. The myth was exacting. At the end of her work, after much practice in her wholeness, she brought the winged horse to each of the miniatures that had carried her forward. Pegasus named each of them. "Now you have a new name. You are strong."

I see a path that the children's works have laid out. It is so crucial that we play therapists understand the layers of what is meant by child development. There is mastery of walking, talking, toilet training, holding scissors. There is the internal growth of the child from absolute dependency to relational interdependency. There is systems awareness of what roles the child carries in the larger family system, and how the child's internal development ingests the family system and its importance. Hardest to reveal and narrate is this holistic self of the child. How is the child perceiving relationship and his place within it? What registers in the child's own implicit world of felt reality, that may or may not be objectively what happened? Nonetheless, it is what happened within the child's self.

This interior meaning-maker is the one who shows up in conversation that may not gel with rational reality and in behaviors that seem to have no reason. These are the realities the child brings into the playroom environment that make use of the child's own organic style of communication. With the tools for metaphor and story, the child lets us enter their own implicit understandings of themselves and those they love. When the child experiences the resonance of being found, and that in this find there is no effort to remake the child's perceptions, then healing is possible.

Epilogue Rose: Remembering One's Self

Rose was 5 years old when I met her. She was the eldest of 3 children, and both parents were very involved in her life. Their concern was in Rose's spaciness, her lack of motivation to pay close attention to her friends during play dates, and her serious focus on imaginary friends. In the parents' cognizance of developmental phases, Rose was not leaving a younger stage soon enough.

Rose took to the sand and its miniatures. Her work seemed easy for her, as it was able to narrate where she spent a good deal of her waking hours. I sensed her relief at having a way in which to create her interior dreams and stories and make them real to someone else. Birds were an area of delight for her. While out on her play equipment outdoors, Rose had evidently spent much time listening to the prattle and watching the speed of birds in her back yard. She had early on described this back yard in great detail. Now, in the tray, she used birds as a strong image to relate her own chirping reality, a reality of untold stories. The birds, with their interactions, their needs and their bird-solutions, reflected Rose's own powerful imagination. Rose told me that when she was swinging on her swing, she was pretty close to what she felt the birds experienced in their flights. She paid attention to those friends and the feelings she gave to them, examining an inner world that had been nearly impossible for her to narrate. The toys narrated this world, becoming real and fluid in the space between us.

What had been building, it seemed, was a growing distance between her young self's great imagination and the need in her parents to speed her up, to let go of this internal world in order to prepare for school demands. Rose's motivation in figuring out how to write her name, chirp back alphabet letters and rote numbers, was eclipsed by this thriving imagination, this sense of wonder.

The Child's Claimed Self

In fact, what Rose taught reveals the wisdom of so many children. When Rose had gathered enough of her own stories, like pinfeathers that would keep her imagination aloft while not flying away, we began our closure. Rose was now 6 years old.

Rose takes many animals and birds, one by one, and flies them from the shelf to the tray. They arrive and settle themselves in a circle. As they come into the tray, Rose gives them each a voice. Rose tells me, "They didn't have a voice. Now they get their voices. They each have to tell their stories. They will tell each other in this circle. They come from an ancient world, and they got here on a big ship. The ship flew through the air from far away. You and me knew some of the people then. But it was really ancient."

"After they tell their stories, then they can remember where they came from. It was way before you and me, a long, long time ago."

The animals whisper. I cannot hear what Rose is having them tell one another. I wait, knowing that these animals are performing their summary task in her behalf. After the story-telling between them, the animals, one by one, fly silently and gently back to their places on the shelves.

Epilogue Rose: Remembering One's Self

Then Rose turns to me. She solemnly tells me, "I will need to forget all this for a long time. To when I'm really old."

I wait, hoping for more understanding. I say, "For how long?"

"I think maybe when I'm 19."

I exhale, knowing that this is very likely. Rose will tuck her imagination safely into a kind of cocoon, using it when it is handy as she grows the ability to carry such a great interior resource into the world.

I often think about what those animals all had to say to one another, to find their stories, and then to be the tribe of animals that would hold space, a great circle, that kept Rose's imagination held within her while she grew up. Is that not what is required, after all? Someone comprehending the wide internal world of each child, in order that that child can figure out how to tuck it in enough so that it does not fly away? But neither does it hold court during the long developmental road of ego-building and social development. When this effort is not understood, when in fact it may be intruded, pushed aside, or broken down through neglect, it is still a world whispering inside the child. It might bring healing to the front. It might believe in a relationship again, using the midwifery of therapy and play to reestablish its presence. Having recovered this interior place, some trust in the core of the child returns.

If we can understand this effort, we will be doing our job. We will wait it out as the child creates voices that hang in there, valued simply for their presences and held in the interior. These stories and voices are not meant to be brought out to the harsher light of reason for interpretation. They bring about their own trust, which comes to us from within the child. And then, it is this trust that moves the child toward individuation and self-esteem, toward a personal voice that knows about itself, that steps into becoming an adult capable of using the talents that have been safely housed in the self of the child.

References

Adams, K, (1999). The Power of Sandplay. *Journal of sandplay therapy,* volume VIII, (2), 89-100.

Alvarado, L. (1991). *Psychology, astrology, and western magic.* Liewellyn Publications.

American Heritage Dictionary. (1992). Third Edition. Houghton Mifflin Co.

Ammann, R. (1991). *Healing and transformation in sandplay.* Open Court.

Ayto, J. (1990). *Arcade dictionary of word origins.* Arcade Publishing.

Badenoch, B. (2008). *Being a brain-wise therapist.* WW Norton And Co.

Baradon, T. (2010). *Relational trauma in infancy: psychoanalytic, attachment and neuropsychological contributions to parent-infant psychotherapy.* Routledge.

Benjamin, J. (2018). *Recognition theory, intersubjectivity and the third.* Routledge.

Benjamin, J. (1988). *The bonds of love.* Pantheon Books.

Bernstein, J. (2005). *Living in the borderland.* Routledge.

Bollas, C. (1987). *The shadow of the object.* Columbia University Press.

Breger, L. (1974). *From instinct to identity: The development of personality.* Prentice Hall.

Bromberg, P. (2011). *Awakening the dreamer*. Routledge.

Bromberg, P. (2011). *The shadow of the tsunami*. Routledge.

Bromberg, P. (2001). *Standing in the spaces*. The Analytic Press.

Churchill, N. (2021). *Journey to Snakewoman*. Dancing Raven Press.

Crittenden, P. (2008). *Raising parents*. William Publishers.

Cunningham, L. (2009). "Approach to the numinous in sandplay: A bridge to creativity." *Journal of Sandplay Therapy*, V18 (2).

Delahooke, M. (2019). *Beyond behaviors*. PESI Publishing and Media.

De Vries, A. (1984). *Dictionary of symbols and imagery*. N. Holland Publishing Company.

Edinger, E, (1985). *Anatomy of the psyche*. Open Court Books, Ltd.

Fernyhough, C. (2012). *Pieces of light*. Profile Books, Ltd.

Flynn, K. (1991). *Making meaning*. Thesis Project, unpublished paper.

Howe, L. (2016). *War of the ancient dragon*. Fisher King Press.

Jung, CG. (1970). *Mysterium coniunctionis in Vol.14 of the collected works*. Princeton University Press.

Kalsched, D. (2013). *Trauma and the soul.* Routledge.

Kalsched, D. (1996). *The inner world of trauma: archetypal defenses of the personal spirit*. Routledge.

Kendler, M. (2017). Must theseus kill the minotaur? coping with destructive aggressiveness in sandplay therapy. *Journal of Sandplay Therapy*, V 26(2).

Mahler, M. (1975). *The psychological birth of the human infant.* Basic Books.

Macnamara, D. (2006). *Rest, play, grow: making sense of preschoolers*. Aona Books.

Neumann, E. (1973). *The child.* GP Putnam's Sons.

References

Pearce, JC. (1977). *Magical child.* EP Dutton.

Peterson, K. (2014). *Helping them heal.* Gryphon House Inc.

Radomsky, L. (2019). *Where dreams come alive.* Chiron Publications.

Raff, J. (2000). *Jung and the alchemical imagination.* Nicolas-Hays Inc.

Samuels, A. (1988). *Jung and the post-jungians.* Routledge.

Schore, A. (2003). *Affect regulation and the repair of the self.* WW Norton & Co.

Siegel, D. (2017). *Mind.* WW Norton & Co.

Siegel, D & Bryson, T. (2021). *The power of showing up: how parental presence shapes who our kids become and how their brains get wired.* Ballantine Books.

Slade, A.& Wolf, D.P. (1994). *Children at play.* Oxford University Press.

Stein, J. (Ed. In Chief). (1975). *The random house college dictionary, revised.* Random House.

Stein, M. Ed. (1982). *Jungian analysis.* Open Court.

Stern, D. (1995). *The motherhood constellation.* Basic Books.

Tustin, F. (2003). *Autistic states in children.* Routledge.

Ulanov, A.B. (2017). *The psychoid, soul and psyche: piercing space-time barriers.* Daimon Verlag.

Ulanov, A.B. (2013). *Madness and creativity.* Texas A & M University Press.

Ulanov, A.B. (2007). *The unshuttered heart.* Abington Press.

Winnicott, D.W. (1971). *Playing and reality.* Routledge.

Winter, R. (1999). Sandplay and Ego Development. *Journal of Sandplay Therapy.* V VIII (1).

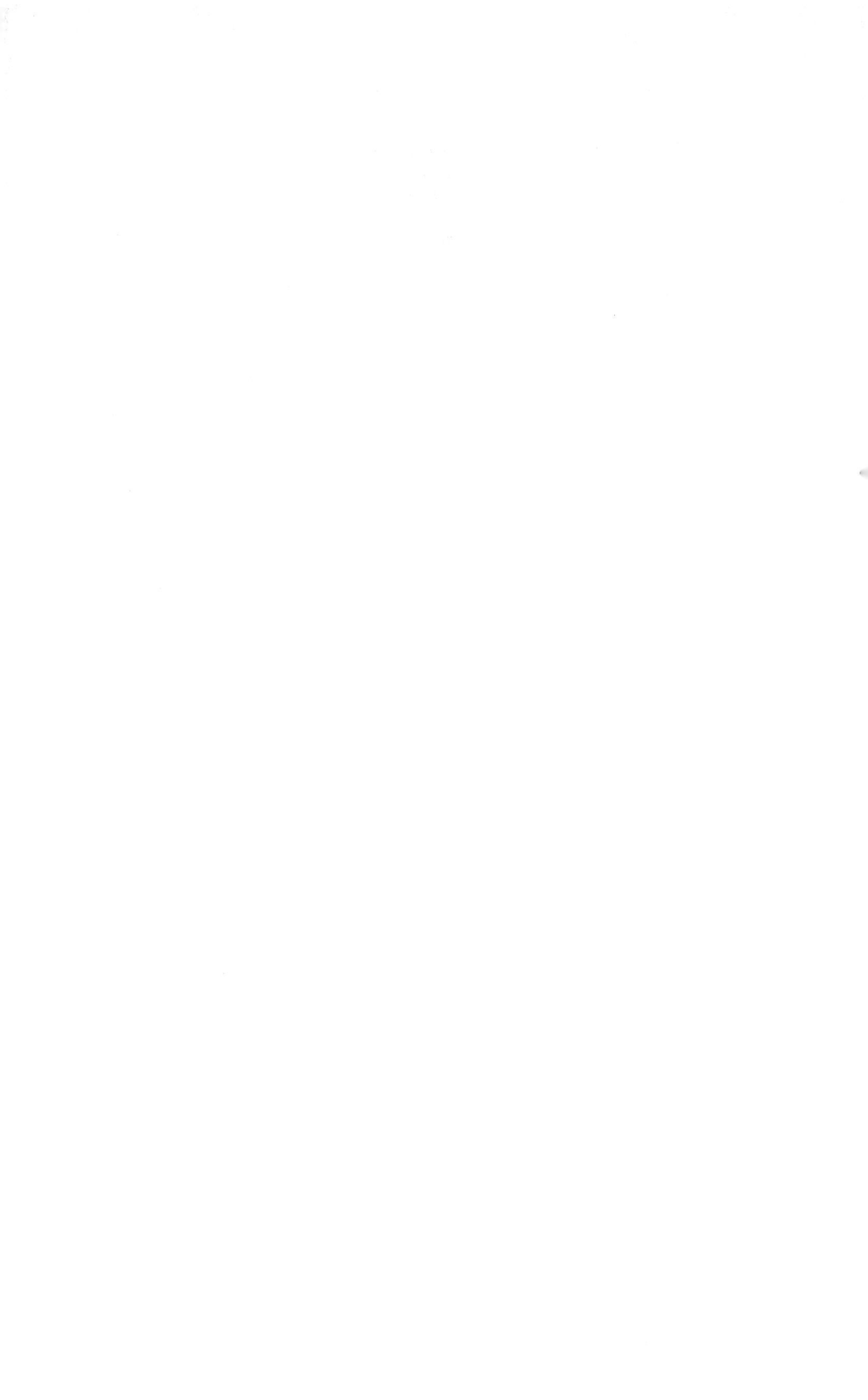

Index

Addiction 135, 156, 242
Adoption 129
Aggression 7, 24, 40, 46, 67, 72, 75, 76, 80–82, 84, 163, 164, 166, 170, 174, 190, 206, 208, 210, 215, 220, 224, 227, 239, 243
Alchemy 10
    Dragon 223
    Gold 215
    Meaning of 214
    Salt 225
Attachment 4, 16, 18, 28, 29, 34–40, 46, 52, 55, 57, 62, 73, 74, 92, 106, 154, 157, 163, 167, 207, 219, 231, 236, 240, 242–244, 251, 272, 278, 291
    Intermittent 45
    Right brain to right brain 95
Autistic diagnosis 90, 129, 130, 135, 138, 145, 245

Being found ix, 54, 57, 59, 63, 71, 106, 120, 129, 131, 133, 135, 137, 139, 141, 143, 145, 253, 271, 284, 286
Benjamin, Jessica x, 19, 21, 132, 133, 183, 184, 197, 291
Brain 8, 25–30, 32–37, 52, 70–72, 85, 108, 118, 121, 132, 159, 174, 222, 229, 250, 258, 260
    Left brain 26, 32, 33, 232
    Limbic system 4–5, 25–27, 35, 44–46, 51, 63–64, 67–70, 157, 169
    gifts of 67
    Neurology of 17–18, 21, 29, 30, 32, 34, 45, 82, 105, 108, 136, 140, 145, 242

relationship 26–27
Right Brain 95, 103, 114, 119, 123, 189, 261, 266, 272, 277
Wiring and firing 18

Children, ix, x, 1–5, 7, 9–11, 16–19, 26, 28, 30, 33, 34, 36–39, 41, 43–47, 53, 55–58, 69, 73, 85, 86, 88, 90, 296
    91, 98, 101, 104, 106–110, 112–114, 117–121, 123, 124, 127, 128, 131, 137–139, 146, 151, 158, 166, 171, 178, 187, 200, 202, 203, 206, 212, 214, 216, 230, 234, 236, 240–244, 250, 251, 253, 255, 259, 262, 264–266, 270–274, 277, 281, 287, 293
    Adopted 27, 46–47, 54–55, 61, 79, 125, 129, 145, 242
    born addicted 134, 135, 242, 243
    child's pace 175, 189, 195
    Child's voices 126, 180, 208, 238, 288, 289
    Claimed self 288, 289
    wiring up 2, 18, 19, 49, 64, 72-73, 80, 133, 154, 189, 272

Death/loss 19, 29, 111–113, 120, 218, 229, 245, 248–250
Dependency 6, 9, 34, 37, 38, 62, 104, 137, 144, 146, 167, 179, 216, 218, 233, 261, 285
    Toward safety 15
Development
    As internal drive 89
    Of safety 3–7, 18, 33–35, 52, 58, 61–63, 65–67, 69–71, 74, 76, 84, 86, 88–90, 92, 95, 97, 99, 105, 109, 114, 118, 120, 121, 134, 138, 147, 148, 151, 158, 174, 204, 214, 248, 251, 275, 285, 289, 291, 293
Diagnoses 167, 183, 269
    Autistic spectrum 129, 245
    Depression 20, 22, 24, 29, 90, 207, 210, 218, 219, 229, 231, 250
    Failure to thrive 137, 157, 242
    Pervasive Developmental Disorder 131
    Selective Mutism 20, 164
Embodiment 27, 41, 65, 66, 145, 174, 262

Failure to thrive 137, 157, 242
Fantasy 45, 49, 80, 101, 105, 154, 210, 244
Feeling states 5, 10, 28, 34, 44, 50, 52, 57–59, 63, 64, 68, 72–74,

Index

79, 83, 106, 110, 134, 151, 160, 161, 184, 185, 207, 214, 217, 227, 231, 237, 272, 279
Filters 96, 262, 272
Fisher king 222
    Holy Grail 223, 227
Freeze pattern 136

Grief 80, 110-114, 193

Healing 9, 10, 18, 25, 37, 44, 92, 107, 144, 146, 150, 153, 161, 175, 179, 180, 196, 198, 202, 216, 227, 233, 237, 244, 249, 264, 269, 271, 273–275, 280, 285, 286, 289, 291
    From the interior 133
    Re-uniting 'you' and 'me' 134
    Use of relationship, in 52

Imagination 5, 10, 32, 57, 59, 70, 80, 82, 97, 99, 101, 102, 104, 120, 143, 145, 148, 154, 155, 172, 174, 185, 190, 192, 201, 203, 204, 210, 214, 218, 223–225, 233, 238, 248, 250, 251, 253–258, 260–266, 279, 287–289, 293
    As access to unconscious 262
Individuation 62, 76, 85, 214, 217, 289
Intelligence 5, 28, 33, 41, 43, 90, 91, 100, 142, 219, 248, 258, 278
    Premature use as defense

Language 1, 3, 4, 9, 16, 17, 19, 22, 26, 27, 31, 33, 41, 43, 52, 56–58, 61, 63, 71–74, 91, 96, 97, 108, 110, 113, 120, 124, 127, 132, 133, 137, 165, 170, 172–174, 177, 178, 200, 201, 203, 238, 239, 246, 249, 254, 255, 257, 261, 273, 275

Memory 11, 27, 39, 43–49, 51, 54–59, 63, 66, 72, 77, 81, 103, 104, 106–113, 114, 118, 122, 124, 126, 132, 143, 151, 157, 160, 161, 168, 169, 173–175, 179, 184–187, 233 , 239, 252, 255, 260, 282, 284
    And relationship 109
    Development of 110
    Explicit, procedural 8

297

Implicit reality 4, 52, 106, 113, 121, 170, 184, 189, 201, 264
   Stored feeling states 134
Meta-communication 197
Mirroring 6, 15, 74, 135, 151, 237, 261
Mutual field x, 70, 133, 153, 161, 171–172, 188, 219, 233, 247, 262–263, 271, 275
   Mutual recognition 8, 132–133, 261
   Mutual space 10, 70, 144, 184, 187, 236, 246

Narration 3, 5, 8, 18, 31, 36, 63, 65, 79, 98, 121, 122, 130, 141, 148, 153, 162, 186
Neglect 19, 47, 55, 57, 73, 88, 132, 133, 135, 137, 138, 147, 158, 164, 165, 167, 172, 174, 289

Parent 7, 16, 18, 19, 21, 31, 36, 37, 45, 46, 56, 58, 65–68, 72–75, 78, 79, 84, 85, 88, 96, 98, 103–105, 108–110, 118, 121, 122, 132, 134, 135, 138, 148, 153, 154, 158, 167, 179, 195, 196, 204, 207, 214, 241, 244, 253, 255, 258, 259, 262, 266, 279, 282, 283, 296
   As regulator 104
   Consultations 218-218
   Parent-child fused states 245
Play Therapy ix, 47, 62, 69, 104, 121, 134, 147, 155–157, 163, 164, 184, 202, 219, 271
   Limitations 240–241
   Stages of treatment 117–180
   Themes 11, 81, 149, 151, 175, 205–206, 209, 211–212, 230
   Treatment Plan 24–25, 160, 233, 246
Power struggle 61, 127, 128, 169

Relationship 2, 6, 7–12, 15, 16, 18–21, 23–26, 29–32, 34, 36, 38–41, 44, 49, 50, 52–57, 59, 62, 64, 65, 67–69, 71, 75, 76, 82, 84, 91, 94, 100, 102, 105, 106, 108, 109, 111–113, 118, 119, 121–123, 133, 134, 136, 138, 148, 150–154, 156, 157, 160–162, 167–169, 172, 174–176, 179, 180, 184–186, 188, 195, 198, 201, 202, 210, 215, 217, 222, 225, 227, 231–233, 237–239,

Index

242, 244, 247, 249, 253–255, 257, 261, 263, 264, 269–272, 278–285, 289
Remembering 39–40, 43, 56–57, 59, 104, 110–111, 114, 168, 190, 194, 253, 264–266
Rituals 48, 55, 110, 143, 206, 212, 223, 265

Schore, Allen 65, 169, 219
Self
    Defended 90, 103
    Of the child 7, 62, 79, 83, 104–105, 114, 151, 201, 235, 251, 255, 285, 289
    Prerequisites 87
Supervision 24, 269, 270, 271–276, 278, 280, 282, 283
    As co-regulator 275–277
    Enactment 189, 220, 280
    False knowing 279–281
    In transference 95, 181–266
    Our own work 95, 234, 249, 274

The between location 22–25
Therapist 1–3, 5, 7, 10–12, 15, 22, 25, 47, 49, 51–53, 55, 58, 92, 109, 110, 118, 121–123, 134, 148–153, 155, 158, 160, 162, 170, 171, 173, 175, 176, 180, 183–185, 187–189, 192, 195, 198, 201–203, 205, 212, 222, 233–235, 238, 239, 241, 255, 257, 259–262, 264, 265, 271–283, 291
    Assignments 153, 263–264
    Concerns of 217
    Empathy 189, 234–235, 249, 252
    Faith in child 59, 213, 226, 266, 274, 280
    Self work 234–236
    Wounds, therapist's 249–250
Transference
    Co-transference 6, 10, 152, 183–185, 187, 202, 229, 231, 233–236, 249, 254, 262, 264, 273, 277, 281
    Dangers of 188
Transitional object 101

Trauma 3–6, 7, 19, 36, 48, 68, 79, 97–98, 101, 125, 129, 135–137, 139, 156–159, 161, 167, 169, 174, 187, 195, 230, 233, 248–249
    Preverbal memory 87, 93, 109, 237
Trust
    Compromised 129–132, 134
    Core 70, 212
    Reciprocity 64

Winnicott x, 57, 62, 66, 68, 71, 101, 132, 144, 161, 162, 219, 270, 293

Printed in the USA
CPSIA information can be obtained
at www.ICGtesting.com
LVHW041751101223
766127LV00010B/342